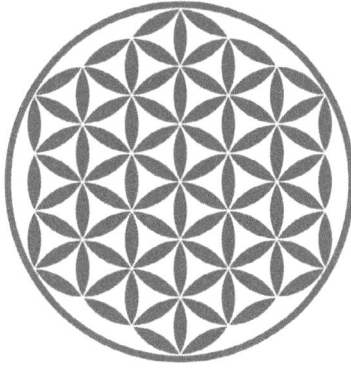

YOU GOT THIS

HOW TO WEAN OFF OPIOIDS, STREET DRUGS AND PRESCRIPTION
MEDICATION WITH LITTLE TO NO WITHDRAWAL SYMPTOMS

DAN KNUDSEN

Author contact information:
Dan Knudsen
4-1104 Kuhio Hwy. # 163
Kapaa, Hawaii, 96746

Library of Congress Control Number: 2019905665

ISBN 978-1-7335354-0-3

First printing 2019
Book design by Najdan Mancic, Iskon Design

DEDICATION

This self-help manual is dedicated to those who are motivated to wean off an addiction, to the thousands of people who have lost their lives because of addiction and to the thousands of people who have lost a family member or a loved one because of addiction.

May they never be forgotten.

TABLE OF CONTENTS

ACKNOWLEDGMENT

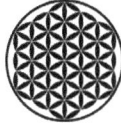

Much love and special thanks to: Carmen Tina Lyman, Gwen Margolis and Ron Margolis for editing, Najdan Mancic, Iskon Design inc. for creating book cover and helping with formatting. Thank you to my dear family and all who have served to make this self-help book available to you.

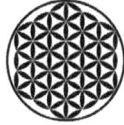

K ratom had been around for many years, but its introduction to western societies has been relatively recent. While it is a naturally occurring biologic medicine, like a new pharmacologic agent, it requires continued research to determine its efficacy, dosage and scheduling, therapeutic index, contraindications, as well as potential side effects and overall safety. Because it comes from a plant, the concentration and molecular characteristics of its active alkaloids can vary from strain to strain, depending on such geologic and geographic factors as soil, composition, available sunlight, water and other variables. Thus, before being introduced into a patient's body, dosages need to be standardized to determine maximum efficacy as well as purity of the product. Additionally, as with any drug or pharmaceutical agent, synthesized or naturally occurring, it is always wise to start with the minimal amount that is required to realize its desired effect. While too high a dosage can cause problems, whereas too little may not be enough to be effective, finding the right dosage needs to be tailored to the needs of each individual. Often, this requires a delicate balancing act between both the art as well as the science of medicine.

All that being said, thus far, from what have been published and studied Kratom holds a real promise as a viable and effective solution to the growing opioid epidemic that is sweeping across America and elsewhere in the western world.

I applaud Dan Knudsen's book and the author's efforts to offer a promising new solution to this destructive, devastating problem, which is leaving behind a shattering wake of death and destruction for countless individuals, families, and communities around the world.

—Arthur Brownstein, M.D., M.P.H., F.A.C.P.M.

Staff Physician
Hale Lea Medical Clinic
Kilauea, HI, 96754
USA

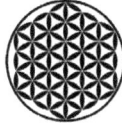

I am not a medical doctor, so I don't give medical advice. This is a self-help manual to wean off opiates, street drugs, and prescription medications. It is not intended to diagnose people and, like many other natural products, Kratom (Mitragyna Speciosa) mentioned in this book is not yet FDA approved, which, makes Kratom not really approved for human consumption. Ordinary people who suffer want to read anecdotes and testimonials on the herbal supplement, natural Kratom leaf powder, and about the various ways it has helped other people.

The scientific community wants to see scientific research. The FDA claims, that Kratom has no medicinal value and, therefore, does not merit approval. Currently, only a few scientific studies have been done on kratom, but the anecdotes and testimonials number in the many thousands. The anecdotal evidence indicates, that natural Kratom leaf powder is an effective herbal supplement, and forthcoming scientific research will prove this fact.

It is quite a paradox because Kratom has been used by millions of people all over Asia and for several centuries for its profound qualities such as natural painkilling, improving focus and cognitive enhancement, reducing withdrawal symptoms and cravings, reducing depression, reducing anxiety, reducing panic attacks, mood enhancing, reduces inflammation in the body including in the arteries and blood vessels, reduces diarrhea, helps regulate glucose and insulin, it can be energetic or deeply relaxing and for many people it improves their sleep but Kratom cannot cure any disease.

Kratom is legal in 46 states in the United States, is currently under observation, which is a bit absurd since it is estimated a couple of million Americans over the last decade have used it and were able to either wean off opiates, street drugs or various prescription medications for depression, anxiety or panic attack, or for chronic pain, in a responsible way to reduce or replace some medications.

Because Kratom is currently not approved for human consumption, I cannot say you should take Kratom. I want you to consider and reflect upon what can happen if you follow the possible guidelines and research it yourself, so Kratom and the information suggested in this self-help manual is for research purposes only, just like all the other people who have done so in the past. I am not responsible for what and how researchers choose to use the suggested information provided.

This self-help manual is basically based on real people's testimonials, sharing's and good advice. They are personal experiences from me and other former or current Kratom researchers. The testimonials are used because these people have weaned off various drugs and gotten their lives back, have happy families again, have become better parents, better employees, got a job or started an education, and for sure increased their quality of life. They got their life back. Read the testimonials over and over again, if you are to become a former addict or ex-user. These testimonials are your stepping stones to freedom and getting your life back.

Most researchers in this book are ordinary people, who don't want to be recognized due to the stigma related to the use of legal/illegal drugs. Many family members, friends and work relations have no idea that people close to them have been using drugs or prescription medication for whatever reason. They have kept it secret from those close to them because of the very strong stigma "People who use drugs have chosen it themselves and they are losers at the bottom of society and they are trash". This stigma is as far from the truth as can be and I will explain this later.

Nevertheless, these people have walked the path before you, they have done it and so can you. Researchers, you know who you are. People who can wean off addictions to opiates, street drugs, and prescription medications are big heroes. Thank you for sharing your personal experiences and advice. I love you and so do all the people who will survive and improve their life and get a second chance for a new life.

If you want to wean off opiates, street drugs and prescription medications, have chronic pain, or are new to the Kratom universe and just want to research something, then this self-help manual might end up being your BFF, Best Friend Forever. It is worth reading everything in here again and again. It is very valuable information on Kratom, detox, vitamins, minerals and coping strategies for anxiety and depression which can help and support you a lot, save your life, your family or a loved one, especially if you are actively using, addicted or a family member is.

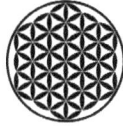

s there an answer to the Opioid, street drug, and prescription medication epidemic and suicide epidemic? Yes, there is an answer. People have successfully weaned off addictions to Opioids, street drugs, Benzodiazepines, SSRIs, AEDs and alcohol with Kratom. This is exactly what this manual is about.

- Kratom can eliminate cravings and withdrawal symptoms
- Rebalance dopamine, serotonin and endorphins
- How to replenish the body naturally with vitamins and minerals
- Information on how to detox the body
- Coping strategies for anxiety and depression

This self-help manual is written to help people wean off mild and moderate drug and alcohol addictions, people who are motivated to wean off but can't because of cravings and repetitive withdrawal symptoms. Kratom does NOT cure anything. Kratom can possibly reduce withdrawal symptoms, reduce anxiety, panic attacks and depressive thoughts, induce energy and clear thinking. There are millions of people who have chronic pain. For those with chronic pain who want to reduce or replace some of their prescription medications due to side effects, in a responsible way, later in the book/manual I go further in depth and describe Kratom, its benefits, how to take it, recipes, potentiators, how to avoid tolerance building up, and how to reduce cravings and withdrawal symptoms. Kratom is not a "one size fits all" substance. We are all built with different, height, weight, diet history, vitamin deficiencies, and we metabolize differently. For some people, Kratom doesn't work as they expected, but maybe they did not have the information they needed when they had the Kratom. Far, far more people have had success with Kratom than those who haven't. You just have to try Kratom to figure out if, and what works for you. Reducing cravings and withdrawal symptoms with Kratom is one thing, this manual also describes how to detox, how to rebalance dopamine, serotonin, and endorphins naturally, how to replenish the body with vitamins and minerals, and natural techniques on how to cope with anxiety, panic attacks, and depressive thoughts without using medication.

Take your time to study this manual. Then, if you decide to, you can use the inspiration and tools given, and should fully be able to successfully reap the benefits.

> *"I have lost 100 lbs. quit taking all the medication I was on 16 different medications and I quit smoking and drinking. I take Kratom every day. I'm so thankful for this plant, I feel amazing and strong. Addiction no longer controls my life."* (DA).

"I love how Kratom takes away my cravings for everything from pain meds to cigarettes and yes, marijuana even! I also forget to take my second dose of Adderall at least half of the time." (FJ).

"I was an IV heroin and meth addict and smoking K2 was worse than those. I got addicted to it almost right away... But Kratom has changed all that. I thought I'd never be able to live even without cannabis, but I don't want it or even like it when I do smoke." (MT).

"I gave up Klonopins after 40 years, thanks to Kratom. Flushed my last script. No more desire." (AL).

"I had to withdraw from Fentanyl patches after being on for 4 years and it was brutal! Lack of sleep nausea and RLS was bad. Then my Doctor recommended Kratom and I took the red strain. (LS).

"I remember when.......when I was a thief... a liar...a cheat.

I remember when my wife couldn't trust me....my behavior was erratic and I couldn't keep a job...I remember when I would suddenly get the flu because I ran out and had to lie because I was supposed to be clean Most of all I remember hating myself and not being able to look at myself in the mirror. I remember the day I discovered Kratom my marriage was just about finished. My wife hated me and I was desperate for a change. I remember all of this every day when I wake up with a smile on my face. Miracles happen every day and Kratom is mine...As long as I remember all of this, I will never believe the lie again." (TV).

"My fiancé has been clean for almost a year off opiates and heroin, over 7 months clean from Suboxone. Thanks to Kratom." (FB).

"Absolutely, I had a 10-year heavy heroin addiction and I am now clean because of Kratom and Kratom only. It just takes away that craving I had. It's amazing. (RJ).

"So, let's be real, I didn't believe in Kratom, I didn't buy all the hype and I was convinced it wouldn't work. So, to prove everyone wrong I got some, then got some more and some more, now fast forward a few weeks and buying pills isn't even a thought anymore, I've had plenty of chances to buy but now I just see it as a waste of money, can't believe after a year of using oxy daily Kratom is what saved me." (MM).

"It's possible, been taking Norco's for at least 11 years. Got some Kratom and haven't touched them the last 8 days and I feel no craving or urge to take any." (LN).

"Day 7 off Fentanyl and oxy, no withdrawals because of Kratom. You have to find the right strain and dose for you. Everybody is different." (SM).

"I was bad on tramadol. I would take 5 at a time. The withdrawal from it was horrible. If you can get a hold of some Kratom, I'd give it a try if I were you. It saved my life." (RS).

"After a few failed attempts to get of Suboxone I quit them cold-turkey with Kratom. Now I don't even take Tylenol now." (JS).

"5 days into detox Methadone, I couldn't have done it without Kratom." (RD).

"All the advice in the world will never help until you are ready to help yourself".....

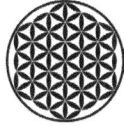

CHAPTER ONE

DRUG-RELATED EPIDEMICS

The Opioid crisis has been raging for decades now. It went from being a crisis into an epidemic. From early on, Vicodin, Oxycodone, Oxycontin and Percocet were meant to be used for the short-term and mostly for cancer patients and the terminally ill. At that time Opioids in general were seen as dangerous and addictive to people.

That changed when one scientific research in 1980 claimed that "Addiction is rare in people treated with Narcotics." (https://www.nejm.org/doi/full/10.1056/NEJMc1700150). Opioids then became mainstream pain medication. Opioid prescriptions were written out left and right. People who used it temporarily ended up becoming addicted and then came back for more pain medication. Millions upon millions of Opioid prescriptions were written out by Doctors who didn't know any better. This scenario went on for many years until the problem was recognized. The federal government began to hit hard on pill mills (doctors who wrote abnormally high numbers of Opioid prescriptions), and Opioid prescriptions in general and people lost legal access to Opioids. Many people ended up on the streets where the illicit supply of Opioids dried out and heroin and prescription medications were the only way to cope with the withdrawal symptoms. Over time heroin has become stronger and stronger, first from being cut with Fentanyl and lately with Carfentanyl which is 10,000 times stronger than morphine. Just a few milligrams are enough to kill an adult. In the last couple years, the number of deaths related to Opioids has skyrocketed.

It is not only Opioids which are of grave concern. We live in an overmedicated society and we may not need all the drugs. Ordinary emotional reactions recently are seen as new psychiatric disorders. People are casually being prescribed psychiatric medications like SSRIs, Benzodiazepines and AEDs. They are all highly addictive or have serious side effects or strong withdrawal symptoms.

What if withdrawal symptoms could be reduced by up to 85% or even more?

Then people who are addicted would be able to wean off drugs by themselves almost for free and still be able to take care of work and family.

Have you ever had the thought that maybe in reality we get really sick when we numb ourselves with drugs? We numb, we get withdrawals, we numb, we get withdrawals, we numb, we get withdrawals. With withdrawal symptoms almost eliminated we have a way out, and we have a path toward recovery and healing.

Then it can lead to a lifestyle change.

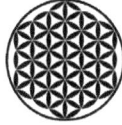

CHAPTER TWO

LOSING FAMILY MEMBERS OR FRIENDS IS A CRUEL REALITY WITH DRUGS

Addiction is very real and it is very intimidating and painful. Never forget that. Addiction destroys families and people lose daughters, sons, moms, dads, cousins, nieces, nephews, uncles, aunties, grandparents and best friends. This is the harsh and tragic reality we need to deal with. It shall never be ignored nor forgotten.

"As I sit and read yet ANOTHER obituary of another addict taken too soon, I think back to the misery of my seventeen years in active addiction: all the times I swallowed 40 perc 10s— vomited them up—and picked them out of my vomit so I wouldn't "waste them." All the times I drove to the dope-man's house with my children in the car and I told them "mommy needs her vitamins." The fear, hurt, and confusion in their eyes should have stopped me, but it didn't. My desire to use was greater than their pain". (YY).

"That makes 15 people now that I have personally lost to heroin. This shit is real people. Everyone's clocks go to zero eventually... when do you want yours to reach its final tick? Think about it... let that sit in...

"I do not want any "I'm sorry" or "my condolences", please. That's not what this is about. Just realize that you will die from it. It is not a matter of if it will kill you or how. It will kill you, it's just a question of when..." (GP).

"I can't post this on open social media because certain family members haven't been notified but my brother has passed away. The police just left my house a little over an hour ago after informing us. This has been my worst fear come true. Please keep my family in your thoughts and prayers. I just can't believe he is gone....." (AJ).

"I'm just trying to get through life the best I can without my boy. I still have a 3 years old son. I've been trying to reach out for all the support I can... I HATE for my 3 years old to see me cry. It scares him. I was 8 months pregnant with him when my oldest died. He was born 5 weeks later, to a broken soul." (CG).

"I have lost 5 people in my life to addiction, 3 to miscarriage." (AS).

"We weren't thinking. Our 4 years old daughter was with an aunt and we figured we could do it one time and then go home and get our daughter that night. It had Fentanyl in it. I pulled over an 8 mile and we split this tiny pack. We both did and next thing I know I wake up in a hospital 2 days *later and the doctor telling me my husband 'didn't make it".* (NK).

"They have no room for all the dead bodies and no beds to help detox. It's no joke people losing their children." (CF).

"I lost my son to drugs in 2009." (PJ).

"Lost my son June 5, 2010. Never gets easier." (RJ).

"Man, I feel your pain. I have lost 7 people this year to Opioids. I am sorry for your loss." (TF).

"Just lost one of my best friends to an overdose. They are going to cut off her life support. It is same day my dad died of an overdose 4 years ago." (TX).

"I'm so, so, sorry for your loss. I have a few friends that also lost children this week. This is why I feel the need to swear. I have 3 boys battling the horrific disease of addiction. All in recovery now, but we know this can change in an instant. Found my son close to death twice. Me and many other addicts' moms wait for that dreaded phone call or knock on the door every day. We have lost 11 of my kids' childhood friends to heroin overdose too. I feel your pain...my heart literally hurts for you. Sending prayers now." (TH).

"My friend's husband lost his battle two nights ago. I'm so sorry for your loss." (AV).

"I'm so sorry for your loss. We lost my uncle to heroin, and it's an awful thing." (BK).

"I am so sorry for your loss. My thoughts and prayers are with you and your family. My cousin lost his 20 years old daughter 6 weeks ago to heroin also." (TH).

"I am so sorry to read this. My son died in March of this year. So, I know the fog you are in... I will send you peace and serenity." (DL).

"I am so sorry. My brother lost his battle in March and my Dad lost his in 2009. It is the hardest way to lose someone ever. Hugs and prayers." (MK).

"I am so very sorry for your loss. Lost my son in January, my only child." (DF).

"I am so sorry, I lost my brother to heroin. I know there are just no words to make you feel better. I am so sorry." (LN).

"Please accept my sincere condolences. I have lost a family member to this and it is devastating." (MO).

"My son lost his battle with heroin." (SD).

"In 2013 my dad died of a heroin overdose. His mom was also an addict. My little sister was on heroin and has been a clean a few months now. My other sister and I are currently in active addiction with pills." (PJ).

"Oh no. I lost a son to heroin." (DM).

"I have a husband, brother, and sister-in-law fighting their battle right now. I'm so scared. I live in fear every second of the day." (CY).

"I am so sorry. Mine, too, is addicted. Love and hugs." (SS).

"So sorry for your loss. I also have a heroin-addicted child and you're always waiting for that call! Sending prayers for strength and healing." (DB).

"As a mother who lost her 24 years old son to an overdose. You need to surround yourself with people that understand addiction and the grief you're experiencing." (LD).

"I hate these days of waking up and learning that another person I know lost their battle! I hate thinking of the pain her child is feeling now that his mommy's gone." (SQ).

"All the times I would be on the floor, my body reeling from all the poison that I had ingested...crawling to the toilet to puke...swearing, 'this is going to be the last time.' I always used the next day. How easily we forget. All the times I spent my last $100 on dope... then had to shoplift food to feed my children. All the times I looked in the mirror and didn't recognize myself. All the times my dad said, with tears in his eyes, 'Please get help. I don't want to bury my child.' This disease is cunning and baffling. I will never forget the misery and hell of my life in active addiction. Never. Ever. I give praise to my Higher Power for helping me out of that pit. But for the grace of God...If you are struggling...never give up trying to get clean. One day you will get there. Just as I did. We DO recover. Carry the hope." (JS).

CHAPTER THREE

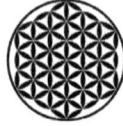

DRUG-RELATED SUICIDE

P eople do not only die from overdoses. Suicide plays a major role in drug-related deaths. People get overwhelmed by their life, the "never-ending withdrawals" and the "no way out" situation they are experiencing.

I personally have lost 8 family members and friends to heroin, prescription medication, alcohol and suicides related to abuse. One hung himself and left his young daughter behind, one used pills in a planned suicide leaving 2 children behind, one shot herself in the head while her 2 children and her husband were in the house. Another one did a planned suicide with heroin. All four above were caught in drug addiction and chose suicide as the way out, the others died prematurely due to addiction and abuse.

"Opiates can kill, even though that is debatable. There are many cases where people can't get treatment and they kill themselves. To me that's the opiate killing U." (Anonymous).

"It's not fair that these drugs are torture and people have no empathy for them when they have no options for treatment. Just to die, is their fate sometimes." (RS).

"This is one of my daughter's friends, addiction was too much. She hung herself." (LN).

When a person choose suicide as an option out of addiction, their children, parents, and loved ones are left behind suffering for the rest of their lives.

If you feel vulnerable and need to talk to someone, you can always call:

National Suicide Prevention Lifeline '1-800-273-8255'

Suicide should never be an option out of addiction.

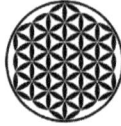

CHAPTER FOUR

STIGMA. IS ADDICTION A DISEASE, A CHOICE OR SOMETHING ELSE?

"**W**hat do you think of when you hear the word "addict?" I think of someone who doesn't take care of themselves appearance/ hygiene wise, someone who steals or prostitute themselves, someone who is homeless." (GC).

"A lot of people today believe that addicts made a choice to become addicted. That's one Stigma I can't stand of our society. It's so ignorant for somebody to think anybody who's addicted to anything, choose that lifestyle." (JS).

"I lost my brother to heroin and I don't find I get any support or understanding. It's terrible. They act like he didn't exist or he wasn't somebody because of the drug. We didn't even know he was using and he was young. It can happen to anyone." (PM).

"I'm sorry for your loss. I know how you feel. I lost my son to pain meds. It's a feeling that no one knows until it happens to them." (PC).

Is addiction a disease, a choice or something else? That is a good question and it needs an answer because many people look down on people who are using prescription medication or street drugs no matter what reason these people may have. Many have such a strong need that they have to get money no matter how. Crime and prostitution are some of the ways, and some end up not being able to take care of themselves, their job or their family, ending up losing it all. Plenty of reasons to stigmatize them and reject them. So, is addiction a disease, a choice or something else?

First of all, some people are ill with chronic diseases and need medication, which is why we have the pharmaceutical industry. People with chronic diseases need some medication to survive.

Then there are people who are predisposed genetically to have a brain imbalance in their chemical composition. They need medication.

Some people end up in tragic accidents, where surgery is lifesaving and may result in a temporary or chronic illness; they need medication too.

Other people end up in situations in their life where they experience things like bad accidents, temporary disease, bankruptcy, sexual abuse, losing a loved one, their job, their house, their company, domestic violence, stress, etc. Some of them choose to numb themselves from their mental or physical pain, trauma or intense emotional experience to survive…. They didn't choose to be addicted; they simply try to survive. For some of the people mentioned above it is a choice to stop when they are motivated enough and have the support they need.

Opioids, street drugs, and prescription medication can be extremely addictive if used over a period of time, some of them over a very short period of time—as little as 2-4 weeks or less. This means that basically anyone using painkillers, SSRIs, Benzodiazepines and AED anticonvulsant prescription medication over a period of time most likely can become addicted. There is one very important thing to take into consideration. People are not necessarily addictive by nature. If so, we would all be addicted to living healthy and only eating a natural diet of vegetables, fruits, fish, nuts, seeds, poultry and meat. Because this is what gives us vitamins, minerals and the real natural dopamine, endorphins and serotonin.

Drugs actually change the brain and that is how and why people become addicted, which is neither a choice or an illness; it is a change in the brain chemistry.

People become addicted because the brain and body change. When taking drugs and experiencing an overflow of dopamine, endorphins and serotonin, the brain will try to balance itself and therefore start to create more receptors to cope with the overflowing neurotransmitters. In a short period of time there are more receiving receptors in the brain. Thus, the new cravings and withdrawals start.

"It isn't always about 'chasing a high'. It's more about not being sick than it is getting high! At the time when I finally quit I was taking 100mg of Hydrocodone at a time and was not getting a high at all!!! But if I didn't take it I would be so sick I was bedridden." (HD).

It is unbearable to observe a loved one addicted to drugs. However, many of us can relate to common behavior, addictions such as: video gaming, shopping, smoking cigarettes, gaining political power, earning money, constantly eating candy and cakes, drinking alcohol, surfing or watching porno, extreme bodybuilding, violent and sadistic behavior, drinking energy drinks, anorexia, bulimia, egoism, constant social media, always taking selfies, seeking likes on Facebook or Instagram, gambling, having plastic surgeries, the list is long… Most of us have experienced the power at least one of these behaviors.

The majority of the people addicted to drugs or medications today are ordinary people; some are wealthy and highly educated with advanced degrees. Some are teenagers at school, young parents, people working as IT engineers, doctors, firefighters, preschool teachers, nurses, self-employed, car washers, company owners, waitresses, senators, politicians, police officers, servicemen and veterans, the unemployed, high school teachers, company board members, movie stars, music stars and sports stars and the list goes on. Addiction doesn't play by any rules, religion, skin color, age, gender or culture. People from all layers of society can become addicted. Famous or unknown, rich or poor. World famous actor Robert Downey Jr. is a good example. Robert Downey Jr. was addicted for years. He almost destroyed his acting career with bad choices and addictions. Robert Downey Jr. is back on track and stronger than ever before, he is now one of the most respected and high paid actors in Hollywood. He is a hero, you can be a hero too.

> *"I can honestly say, that NO ONE would EVER guess in a million years what I do EVERY fucken day! I have a beautiful 4-bedroom home, nice vehicle, all paid for, no debts or payments to make, all name brand clothes for both me and my children, a fridge FULL of organic food, kids get amazing lunches packed for school, hair professionally done etc. List could go on and on! Would have even more going for me, IF, I didn't have a fucken $4000/month habit." (MK).*

People with addictions are everywhere. Actually, some of your family and friends might be addicted and you may not even know it.... We are all in this together. Nobody is better or less than anyone else...... Using a drug, prescription or not, changes the brain chemistry and some users make really bad choices. That behavior is not the original blueprint addicted people were born with.

We should never judge anyone before we have looked at ourselves or walked a mile in their shoes. Let's stop judging and stigmatizing other people. Don't put anyone down, reject or point fingers because of an addiction. We need to have respect, compassion, empathy and help each other. Anyone, anytime, anywhere, under certain circumstances, can end up an addict.

"I've literally known people in their late thirties with great jobs, nice house, nice car, never did drugs before, live in the suburbs who got injured, put on pain pills, then they suddenly got cut off, still had the pain and were withdrawing so they started doing heroin. It's awful" (LA).

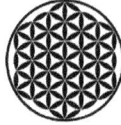

CHAPTER FIVE

THE VICIOUS CYCLE OF DRUGS

"**O**ver 2,000,000 Americans are estimated to be dependent on Opioids and an additional 95,000,000 used prescription painkillers in 2016." (Centers for Disease Control, 2017).

"The estimated number of Opioid overdoses for 2016 is between 59,000 to 65,000 deaths." (Centers for Disease Control, 2017).

There is limited public information available about the extent of the use of psychiatric drugs among the US adult population. The information below is only from the people who reported. Stigma surrounding use of psychiatric drugs leads to underreporting.

"Overall, 16.7% of 242 million US adults reported filling one or more prescriptions for psychiatric drugs in 2013. That included SSRIs, Benzodiazepines, antipsychotics, and those classified as anticonvulsants. (https://jamanetwork.com/journals/jamainternalmedicine/fullarticle/2592697>)

Suicide statistics 201: Each year 44,965 or more Americans die by suicide. Suicide is often drug-related. Stigma surrounding suicide leads to underreporting. (https://afsp.org/about-suicide/suicide-statistics/).

I wonder how high the shadow numbers are and how many people committed suicide beyond of the above numbers, because they ended up in a "no way out of addiction" situation.

Some of the 95,000,000 Americans which temporarily used prescription painkillers will become addicted. 2-4 weeks on prescription painkillers, sometimes less, can make almost anybody addicted and end up in the prescription medication vicious cycle, (I will explain soon in the restless leg syndrome (RLS) example). Some will be able to wean off after a short period of use. The rest who get cut of their access to prescription medication will most possibly go to the streets for their painkillers, or simply change addiction (to avoid withdrawal symptoms), to Heroin, Meth, Fentanyl, Cocaine, Xanax, Valium, methadone, or whatever can eliminate their withdrawal symptoms, their physical, psychological or emotional pain.

Recently new and stronger drugs have hit the streets. These altered and stronger street drugs are a big reason for some of the high numbers of deaths related to opiates. The street drugs are being cut with stronger drugs. Fentanyl is 1000 times stronger than morphine, Carfentanyl 10,000 times stronger than Morphine. (draxe.com 2016).

"How many people are using opiates because they were injured awhile back and they automatically gave you something to alleviate the pain? It's coming up on July 10th and in 1997 when I broke my wrist whilst rollerblading, it will be twenty years of this shit for me. I was started on Lortab then Perfect 5 then 10s then OxyContin 10s then 20s then I was finally on 60mg OxyContin then my insurance wouldn't pay for it so they put me Opana 40mg 3 times a day and Oxycodone 20mg 3 times a day and Klonopin 2 mg twice a day. That's what I'm on now and I want nothing more than to get off this shit. I've tried to go cold turkey, but I didn't have the .... required to go through that hell. So, I ask, what do I do to get off this shit because I'm sick and tired of living like this. It is no life. (DF).

Some street drugs and prescription medications have serious side effects and/or withdrawals symptoms like muscle spasms, involuntary movements and restless legs, etc. which then often require other prescription drugs. One thing leads to/ or replaces another. One street drug or prescription drug has negative effects and another or two prescription medications are needed to alleviate the side effects or withdrawals symptoms of the original drug. Therefore, many street drug users and prescription medication users use several prescription medications legal or illegal, sometimes as many as 5+ different prescription medications.

Restless legs are a very well-known withdrawal symptom and people weaning off drugs suffer immensely from it. Many people who have weaned off drugs say that RLS is the worst withdrawals symptom. RLS in itself can cause insomnia, sleep deprivation, stress, pain, depression, anxiety, nightmares, panic attacks, etc. The medication below is not mentioned here only because of RLS, but because the majority of them are also used to treat sleep problems, anxiety, muscle tension, depression, pain and withdrawal symptoms or side effects from other drugs.

Some RLS prescription medication treatments:

1. **Benzodiazepines**: (Xanax, Klonopin, Valium, Ativan, Restoril, Rohypnol, Librium, Halcion, etc.). Benzodiazepines are widely used in medicine to treat anxiety and insomnia. These are synthetic substances normally seen as pharmaceutically-manufactured tablets, capsules and occasionally as injectables. They act as depressants and sedatives of the central nervous system (CNS). They do not affect the symptoms of RLS, but they are often used to help patients relax and/or sleep. Benzodiazepines are highly addictive and have serious side effects and serious withdrawal symptoms.

2. **Opioids**: (Norco, Oxycodone, Oxycontin, Vicodin, etc). Opioids are painkillers, sometimes they are used to help relieve RLS symptoms. Opioids are highly addictive and have serious side effects and serious withdrawal symptoms.

3. **Antiepileptic drugs (AEDs)/Anticonvulsants**: (Gabapentin, Lyrica, Neurontin, Clonazepam, Topomax, Horizant, Lamictal, Tegretol, etc. and anti-parkinso-

nians). These drugs are often used for patients suffering from seizures, chronic pain, and neuropathic pain, and epilepsy as well as many other neurological and psychiatric conditions. They are widely prescribed for many things. 100 people overdosed on "Gabapentin" in West Virginia in 2016. (DoctorsTv.com). Very often they are used to reduce withdrawals from other drugs. Not addictive, but the withdrawals are very painful. Which keeps people on it, or make people use other prescription medications to cope with the very painful withdrawals symptoms. Anticonvulsants are highly addictive and have serious side effects.

A new study shows that Gabapentin and Lyrica are causing the brain to decline because they block the formation of new brain synapses. Warner-Lambert and Pfizer have been fined upwards of a billion dollars for off-label marketing. It causes the brain to decline faster than any substance known to man. (Medicalhealthnow.info).

Several anticonvulsant medications are recognized as mood stabilizers to treat or prevent mood episodes in bipolar disorder. Some even for anxiety, depression, fibromyalgia, migraines, ADHD, or weight control. (Source. European Monitoring Center for Drugs and Drug Addiction).

The paradox here is that many street drugs and prescription medication side effects will make people experience RLS, anxiety, uncontrollable movements, depression, panic attacks and/or weight gain or weight loss, etc. and therefore tend to increase the use of many other prescription medications.

The 3 RLS treatments above have several things in common:

- They can be very addictive.
- They're unnatural, synthetic pharmaceutical drugs.
- They're expensive.
- They all come with serious side-effects.
- They have some very nasty withdrawal symptoms.

Antiepileptic drugs (AEDs)/anticonvulsants, increase the risk of suicidal thoughts or behavior in patients taking these drugs for any indication. (John P. Cunha, DO, Facoep. and Rxlist. com 2017).

"I am horribly addicted to Gabapentin. They gave it to me while detoxing from Xanax. This is by far 10 times harder to get off." (LJ).

"I was a closet Xanax and Adderall abuser. Now trying to get off Percocet's. I also am addicted to Gabapentin." (JL).

"I'm withdrawing from Lyrica and it's awful. I was using Ativan to help, and now I'm withdrawing from that as well. In the past I've came off Opioids." (TO).

4. **SSRI, (Selective serotonin uptake inhibitors)**: (Celexa, Lexapro, Prozac, Luvox, Paxil, Zoloft, etc). SSNRI and SSRI medication is used to treat depression, anxiety and mood disorders.

SSRI medications are often being used to treat side effects or withdrawal symptoms on the 3 RLS treatment medications above. These medications are very often linked together in various ways of multiple drug use.

"I feel like there is no cure for restless legs besides dope. Which happens to also be what caused it." (MS).

This is just a silly example to point out what I mean: One Opioid detox withdrawals symptom is restless legs. (Gabapentin to fix the restless legs), Depression from Gabapentin, (Celexa to fix the depression from Gabapentin), Insomnia from Celexa. (Xanax to fix the insomnia from Celexa).....

"Is it bad to take Gabapentin and Xanax together for the withdrawals from Suboxone?" (RA).

The different opioids, street drugs, and prescription medications have so many side effects and withdrawal symptoms that they keep overlapping each other, and many medication/drug users often have to be on several prescription medications to even be able to function minimally in our society.

The good news is: Kratom by itself or in combination with DLPA or other over the counter products (more on this ahead), has helped many, many people to wean off from abusing or addictions to several prescription medications, for example by reducing the RLS and the majority of other withdrawal symptoms.

"Kratom helped my RLS enough to let me sleep." (WM).

"I haven't taken Lyrica since I started Kratom. 3-4 weeks now. Withdrawal symptoms were foot pain and restless legs, aches, and pain. Didn't have the pain when taken Kratom." (UP).

"Yes, RLS was the worst part of the withdrawal process for me. I use Kratom. It works absolutely wonderful." (DL).

"Kratom always knocks out RLS for me." (AF).

"A high number of individuals reported successfully using Kratom as a substitute to help abstain from the use of other substances perceived as addictive and/or causing harm. These substances were primarily Opioids, Benzodiazepines, and antidepressants." (Swogger et al 2015).

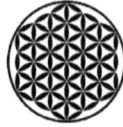

CHAPTER SIX

KRATOM SPECIFICS

Kratom is a tree (Mitragyna Speciosa) in the coffee tree family (Rubiacacia). It is native to Southeast Asia (Indonesia, Thailand, Malaysia, and Papua New Guinea), and it thrives in sub-tropical and tropical regions.

"Kratom is not a drug. Kratom is not an Opiate. Kratom is not a synthetic substance. Naturally occurring Kratom is a safe herbal supplement that's more akin to tea and coffee than any other substance." (americanKratom.org/science).

Kratom in general has been used since at least 1836 in Asia by millions of people for its health qualities and as a herbal supplement. (Reduces pain, reduces withdrawal symptoms, reduces cravings, reduces depression, reduces anxiety, reduces panic attacks, it can be either sedating or energizing, elevating mood, anti-diarrhea, relaxation, enhanced sociability, increased focus and clear thinking, anti-inflammatory, lowers blood pressure, stimulant or analgesic, appetite suppressant, treatment for malaria, cough and fever reduction etc.)

"Results of several analyses published within the past year indicate that large numbers of people are using Kratom for the management of Opioid withdrawal and pain." (Walter C. Prozialeck, Ph.D. 2016).

In Asia the leaves are often chewed to gain the energizing and stimulating effects for hard labor. Kratom is also used to prepare tea or is ingested in powder preparations for its many health benefits.

The leaves contain active compounds, the most known are **Mitragynine and 7-hydroxymitragynine**. There are more than 40 compounds in Kratom leaves. (Shellard 1974, https://www.ncbi.nlm.nih.gov/pubmed/4607551).

"The effects of the main alkaloids, i.e., mitragynine and 7-hydroxymitragynine have mainly been explained by interactions with the Opioid, serotonin and dopamine receptors." (Boyer https://www.ncbi.nlm.nih.gov/pubmed/18482427)

Since Kratom also affects Dopamine and Serotonin receptors it can possibly explain why it can reduce withdrawal symptoms and therefore can help people wean off not only Opioids, but in general street drugs, alcohol and prescription medications like Benzodiazepines and SSRI etc. Throughout this book there will be various reports and testimonies from ordinary people who, by themselves, have used Kratom to wean off illicit use of Opioids, street drugs, alcohol, Benzodiazepines, SSRI medications.

At least 2 scientific studies have demonstrated that mitragynine has an antidepressant effect. (Kumarnsit et al. 2007 and Idayu et al. 2011, Dr. Tom O'Brien).

At least 1 scientific study has demonstrated that Kratom has been used to self-manage alcohol withdrawal symptoms. (Haveman-Reinicke 2011, Dr. Tom O'Brien).

LIST OF ALKALOIDS IN KRATOM, MITRAGYNA SPECIOSA

The concentration percentages listed come from different studies of alkaloid concentrations in Mitragyna speciosa–the Kratom leaf. Some of the alkaloids listed still need to be studied more specifically in order to determine their potential activity.

- **Ajmalicine (Raubasine)**: Cerebrocirculant, antiaggregant, anti-adrenergic (at alpha-1), sedative, anticonvulsant, smooth muscle relaxer. Also found in Rauwolfia serpentina.

- **Akuammigine**: -

- **Ciliaphylline**: antitussive, analgesic. < 1% of total alkaloid content found in Kratom leaf.

- **Corynantheidine**: μ-Opioid antagonist, also found in Yohimbe. < 1% of total alkaloid content found in the Kratom leaf.

- **Corynoxeine**: Calcium channel blocker. < 1% of total alkaloid content found in the Kratom leaf.

- **Corynoxine A and B**: Dopamine mediating anti-locomotives. < 1% of total alkaloid content found in the Kratom leaf.

- **Epicatechin**: Antioxidant, antiaggregant, antibacterial, antidiabetic, antihepatitic, anti-inflammatory, anti-leukemic, antimutagenic, antiperoxidant, antiviral, potential cancer preventative, alpha-amylase inhibitor. Also found in dark chocolate.

- **9-Hydroxycorynantheidine**: Partial Opioid agonist

- **7-hydroxymitragynine:** Analgesic, antitussive, antidiarrheal; primary psychoactive in Kratom, roughly 2% of total alkaloid content found in the Kratom leaf.

- **Isomitraphylline**: Immunostimulant, anti-leukemic. < 1% of total alkaloid content found in the Kratom leaf.

- **Isomitrafoline**: < 1% of total alkaloid content found in the Kratom leaf.

- **Isopteropodine**: Immunostimulant

- **Isorhynchophylline**: Immunostimulant. < 1% of total alkaloid content found in the Kratom leaf.

- **Isospeciofoline**: < 1% of total alkaloid content found in the Kratom leaf.

- **Mitraciliatine**: < 1% of total alkaloid content found in the Kratom leaf.

- **Mitragynine**: Indole alkaloid. Analgesic, antitussive, antidiarrheal, adrenergic, antimalarial, possible psychedelic (5-HT2A) antagonist. Roughly 66% of total alkaloid content found in the Kratom leaf.

- **Mitragynine oxindole B:** < 1% of total alkaloid content found in the Kratom leaf.

- **Mitrafoline**: < 1% of total alkaloid content found in the Kratom leaf.

- **Mitraphylline**: Oxindole alkaloid. Vasodilator, antihypertensive, muscle relaxer, diuretic, anti-amnesic, anti-leukemic, possible immune stimulant. <1% of total alkaloid contents in the Kratom leaf.

- **Mitraversine**: -

- **Paynantheine**: Indole alkaloid. Smooth muscle relaxer. 8.6% to 9% of total alkaloid contents in the Kratom leaf.

- **Rhynchophylline**: Vasodilator, antihypertensive, calcium channel blocker, antiaggregant, anti-inflammatory, antipyretic, anti-arrhythmic, antithelmintic. < 1% of total alkaloid content found in the Kratom leaf.

- **Speciociliatine**: Weak Opioid agonist. 0.8% to 1% of total alkaloid content of the Kratom leaf, unique to Kratom.

- **Speciofoline**: -

- **Speciogynine**: Smooth muscle relaxer. 6.6% to 7% of total alkaloid contents of the Kratom leaf.

- **Speciophylline**: Indole alkaloid. Anti-leukemic. <1% of total alkaloid contents of the Kratom leaf.

- **Stipulatine**:—

- **Tetrahydroalstonine**: Hypoglycemic, anti-adrenergic (at alpha-2)

Many of the secondary chemicals found in Mitragyna Speciosa Kratom are present in small yet appreciable quantities, and their synergetic role and activity in the general pharmacology of Mitragyna speciose, Kratom is not yet fully understood, as thorough research has only just begun. (Justin, 2014. Kratomscience.com).

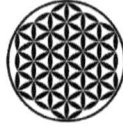

CHAPTER SEVEN

IS KRATOM DANGEROUS?

I n the US, there are an estimated several million users purchasing Kratom products from more than 10,000 retail outlets with estimated annual sales of 207,000,000 dollars (Botanical Education Alliance, 2016).

"Animal studies have demonstrated some signs consistent with physical dependence and withdrawal at what appear to be extraordinarily high dosages of in terms of milligrams. Specifically, laboratory rats were given 30 mg/kg/day, equal to an oral dose of about 990 mg/kg (Yusoff et al., 2016). Humans would need to consume over 600-800 oral doses of Kratom in a single sitting to achieve the same milligram dose. In fact, no evidence has demonstrated the onset of physical dependence and withdrawal at levels consistent with human dosage. However, the modest desirability of the effects would seem to make such a heroic effort extremely unlikely because the pleasure derived from consumption does not appear similar in magnitude to that produced by far less costly and readily available doses of typical substances of abuse including marijuana, alcohol, stimulants, sedatives, and Opioids. The lack of public health problems or abuse is, despite the fact that there has been widespread consumption of Kratom by consumers for more than two decades in the US, and likely consumption among some populations for decades longer. More research is needed to understand the relevance of such findings to human consumption and to better characterize Kratom among other substances." (Dr. Henningfield, 8 Factor analysis 2016).

"Traditional uses are not associated with major toxicity even with chronic uses and there are no observations of dependence or misuse or abuse." (Dr. Oliver Grundman College of Pharmacy, University of Florida 2017).

"As of November 14. 2017, an FDA commissioner made a public announcement that 36 fatalities are associated to Kratom use. However 35 of the fatalities included several multi-drug intoxications." (Dr. Oliver Grundman College of Pharmacy, University of Florida). Multi-drug intoxication is several drugs taken at the same time, such as Opioids, Benzodiazepines, SSRI medications, etc. illicit or prescribed. Jane Babin, Ph.D., in molecular biology recently did an in-depth research on the FDA claims and rejected all of them. (FDA fails to follow the science on Kratom).

"A new review by the American Kratom Association of the FDA Adverse Event Reporting System (FAERS) database shows that, from 2011-2017, not a single death has been attributed solely to Kratom anywhere in the United States." (AmericanKratomAssociation.com).

"Although some cases have been reported of deaths attributed to Kratom use, no solid evidence has yet been provided where the substance was the sole contributor to the fatality." (Warner et al 2016). It is always a good idea to stay away from Kratom with additives. Kratom sold from head shops or gas stations often have additives and these additives can be synthetic. Know your vendor, the best vendors are often American online Web shops. The potency of Kratom often varies from vendor to vendor due to harvest methods, area, mineral content in the dirt and age etc.

"The DEA (Drug Enforcement Administration) argue that Kratom is dangerous because there were 660 calls related to Kratom exposure" from 2010 through 2015, an average of 110 a year. By comparison, exposures involving analgesics accounted for nearly 300,000 calls in 2014, while cosmetics and personal care products, cleaning solutions, antidepressants, and antihistamines each accounted for more than 100,000." (Warner et al 2016, Dr. Tom O'Brien.ie).

The mainstream news is currently spreading misinformation about Kratom.

The pharmaceutical industry may be trying to get Kratom banned through FDA. Strong forces and their very active and wealthy lobbyists are trying to restrict access to Kratom, which it is not surprising because the pharmaceutical industry stands to lose trillions of dollars because people can use Kratom to wean off opioids, prescription medication, maintenance drugs as well as illicit prescription medication sold as street drugs. The pharmaceutical industry created the opioid crisis;

they sell all the maintenance products like methadone and suboxone etc, and they also sell naloxone and the generics for people who overdose... and all the other prescription medications which follow an addiction and the side effects of the side effects... If a person who uses several prescription medications daily or a maintenance drug like Methadone, and decides to wean off the drugs with ease, just like that, then the pharmaceutical industry loses a long-time customer and all the money attached to that person. Now, what if 1,000,000 out of 33,000,000 drug users use Kratom to wean of an addiction?

"I use Kratom daily for pain and anxiety and am functioning much better than I did when taking Fentanyl, Oxycodone, Xanax, Cymbalta, and Abilify so I'm not going back there." (MH).

"Self-treatment of Opioid withdrawal symptoms with Kratom is widely used in Southeast Asia and has been used since the 1950s. Self-treatment of Opioid Withdrawal symptoms with Kratom is currently increasing in the USA. "Kratom can be used as a legal means to treat opiate withdrawal." (Griffen et al. 2016).

Kratom is not a drug. Kratom is not an opiate. Kratom is not a synthetic substance. Kratom, a natural supplement, is well known for centuries in Asian medicine for its painkilling qualities, reducing withdrawal symptoms, anti-inflammation, anti-anxiety, anti-panic, anti-depression, clear thinking, and energetic qualities. Naturally occurring Kratom leaf without additives is a gateway OUT of addiction and it is legal in 44 states. It works. I have met a few people who said, "Yeah, I have tried Kratom in the past and Kratom doesn't work for me." Here are some reasons that may be true:

1. If Kratom is not used correctly, is too old or has additives, it can decrease its effect.

2. If you don't suffer from pain, then you don't experience the painkilling qualities.

3. If you are not weaning off an addiction, then you don't experience the eliminated cravings and withdrawal symptoms.

4. If you are not suffering from depression, and are happy with your daily life, then you don't experience the anti-depressive qualities.

5. If you don't suffer from anxiety, then you don't experience the anti-anxiety qualities.

6. If you don't suffer from panic attacks, then you don't experience the reduced panic attacks.

7. If you don't suffer from lack of energy i.e. fibromyalgia, etc. Then you may not experience the extra energy.

That leaves healthy people with… clear thinking… that is not a high, maybe unless you are writing a dictionary on a foreign language.

Some uneducated people claim that Kratom is a party drug… Party drug? Do they refer to Kratom tea party???

"If you're looking to get high, Kratom won't work. It does not get you high. I think people confuse the "uplifting" feeling you may experience with Kratom with being "high". (ET).

"If you want to get high, Kratom isn't for you. You'll end up puking trying to get high." (JD).

"Makes me nauseated if I take too much...no high...at the right dose I get pain relief and am a bit talkative...that is it...but that is enough..." (KS).

"If you're smoking weed to kill pain or help with anxiety, Kratom can definitely work for you. If you want to get high, you'll be completely wasting your money." (KP).

"If you're looking for a high you're wasting your time and money." (IL).

"No, it doesn't get you high...but you can definitely tell the difference as to why people quit taking pain pills and started Kratom." (KM).

People don't get high on Kratom. Why would anyone ingest something that doesn't give a high, doesn't taste good and may almost make them gag because it is a powder when they can smoke a joint or drink a beer? It doesn't make any sense. So, no. Kratom does not give you a high. BUT, for people who have suffered and been disabled in various degrees by pain, social anxiety, depression, panic attack and lack of energy. They feel relief and that increases their levels of physical activity, family life, social life, new optimistic perspectives on life, or offers a way out of an addiction in drug-hell and it's all-inclusive, they become happy.

Kratom users become parents again, they start working or go back to study again. These positive life-changing experiences will give anyone euphoria, not because of the Kratom itself, but because of the lift in their life quality.

"With the help of Kratom, me and my husband are 90 days clean from a 6-years opiate addiction I never thought I'd ever be able to say that. WOW! and tomorrow this mamma starts college which is another amazing thing I never thought I'd get to say again this is all thanks to Kratom the mood lift energy boost pain relief anxiety control and just all-around great outlook on life I have again." (JH).

"I feel that this wonderful plant we use has helped me go from an overweight, almost 300 lbs alcoholic opiate addict to a 205 pounds laborer with extreme endurance. I simply achieved this by eating healthy foods and only using things like Kratom and only natural alternatives to the things man has messed with. I've totally turned my life around from a very sick man, to a fit 55 years old." (MD).

"My life was hell. Me and husband both had a daily 300mg morphine addiction and now we have been clean almost a year and I graduate college 2018! I owe Kratom everything!" (JN).

"I'm coming off a four-year streak of heavy opiate use (started with Oxy, then heroin become my love) and it's been tough but so far it's fucking worth it! It feels so good to wake up in the morning, put on makeup and go to work and not have to worry about how I'm going to get high to get through the day. We got this shit!" (PB).

If Kratom is used on a daily basis for a long period of time it can be habit-forming and create a normal dependency like everything else. However, withdrawal symptoms happen when dopamine, serotonin and endorphin etc. are out of balance. When natural Kratom leaf powder is used to wean off an addiction it should be tapered down and stopped after the initial withdrawal symptoms which can last a couple months depending of the half life of the drug. The brain receptors need a break; you need healing and natural rebalancing of dopamine, serotonin and endorphin with a healthy diet and exercise. If not, it is most likely you can experience withdrawal symptoms. Why? Not because of the natural herb kratom but simply because your brain receptors didn't get a break, healing and natural rebalancing.

So, get yourself a healthy diet, detox, rebalancing and exercise going on, NOW. If the natural balance is there, health and healing are there. Do the effort and do it now. Just do it.

In this book, Kratom is specifically suggested to be used for a temporary period of time up to some couple of months or so while coping with serious drug cravings and withdrawal and then reduce the use of Kratom. Secondly, it is to reduce prescription medication and cope with chronic pain, depression, and anxiety etc. in a natural and responsible way. If you have an addictive personality, be extra aware and use Kratom in a responsible way.

Adverse reactions which can occur at high doses of Kratom: Nausea, vomiting, increased urination, constipation, itching, loss of appetite, sweating. This is why people can't overdose on Kratom.

Kratom should be used cautiously with patients who have thyroid disorders, liver disorders, gastrointestinal disorder or neurologic disorders. Avoid during pregnancy or lactation and in children due to a lack of available research. (C Ulbricht et al. J Diet Suppl 10 (2), 152-170. 6 2013).

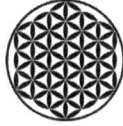

CHAPTER EIGHT

IS KRATOM ADDICTIVE?

The majority of people say that Kratom withdrawals are the same as if you drink coffee daily and then suddenly stop drinking coffee. For most people coffee withdrawals are usually 1-2 days with light headache, little nausea, sweating and tiredness. Kratom is in the coffee family.

Some people say it is addictive. I had a conversation with a person who claimed that Kratom was very addictive and its withdrawals was worse than opiates. She ended up telling me that she only had Kratom from 1 specific street head shop. She said she paid $20 for 1 gram. I asked her if a "bell didn't ring" since 1 oz of Kratom is around 28 grams and usually cost around $8—$10 an oz. Possibly, it was laced with a legal or illegal synthetic drug variation which can both be very addictive and have serious withdrawals. Know your source.

At FlowerOfLife808.com You can find high quality organic natural Kratom leaf powder without additives, tested for salmonella, mold and E-coli etc.

Kratom is a natural plant, Kratom is not synthetic. Kratom is not addictive when used responsibly and Kratom does not have serious withdrawals. A responsible way is, stay away from Kratom with any additives, stay away from super enhanced Kratom. Less Kratom is more and remember to do tolerance breaks which is described later.

"Your body develops some kind of dependency to anything you consume on a daily basis, and when you stop, you will likely experience some symptoms. That is biology." (MK).

Feedback from some Kratom users: "My experience with coming off Kratom: last dose was yesterday. I was scared, my brain telling me it would be painful. I was afraid of.... Nothing. I can barely tell I have not taken it. I have been taken Kratom for 6 months and needed a tolerance reset. When I was weaning off opiates, not using Kratom, I was in so much pain I could barely walk and was deathly sick for over a week. Kratom reset is easier for me than coming off coffee." (AN).

"I used to be on it several times a day and now I take it once and sometimes forget to. I have no withdrawal or problems." (RR).

"I have used Kratom for more than 1 year for insomnia and its anti-anxiety qualities, usually a couple times during the day and in the evening. I have not increased tolerance and I sometimes forget to take it. I usually do a 2 days tolerance break every week. No dependency or withdrawal symptoms of any kind." (DK).

"It is addictive. But as addictive as coffee. No more. And just because something's physically addictive doesn't mean that it is dangerous. Caffeine is physically addictive." (BH).

"I was tired and slept most of the day, that is the worst withdrawals from using up to 30 grams a day (15 teaspoons)". (RC).

"Taper and you'll be fine! Even if you can't taper, it's a very mild withdrawal, NOTHING like an opiate withdrawal. And, you may not have any at all, if you're using smaller doses." (TC).

"It's crazy how everyone is so different. I still tell everyone I know about Kratom because it's amazing! A little withdrawal is fine by me because it got me off Suboxone." (ET).

"Taper down to a 5g dose, most people don't experience any withdrawals at all". (YY).

"I have dosed regularly with just Kratom I've not taken any pain meds. I'm surprised with how minimal the withdrawals are. I'm still shocked that Kratom helped me. I've been through bad withdrawals in the past and not only is Kratom amazing but it's do-able if that makes sense". (LJ).

"I had to quit Kratom to do a surgery. I quit cold turkey and I had no withdrawals. Is my pain back? Yes of course, not more than before. My daily dose was 11/2 tsp 3-4 times daily. In the past I have used Kratom to withdraw from

heavy drugs so I was prepared, but I had no withdrawal. I can't wait to return to my Kratom." (Anonymous).

"So, my Kratom journey has ended. It was very helpful for me, physically I'm feeling better and don't feel I need it anymore. I was also starting to use it a little bit too much. I'm on the 40 hours mark of no Kratom after 4 months of heavy use. Right now, it is just hot and cold sweats and some nausea. I hope this is as bad as it gets". (KD).

"You are going to be fine. Keep telling yourself that. When I quit Kratom after 2 years of using it, I had VERY mild withdrawals symptoms that lasted for a week. Most was just from the fear of what I expected and a lot was just in my mind. At least you are not coming off Methadone or Heroin, etc. Now that's unbearable…." (ZZ).

"I have been on Kratom for 15 years. If you take Kratom that long, or take it longer and often enough, you will experience withdrawals. Are they horrid? Nope, but sure they suck." (CA).

"Nothing compared to Opioids and prescription medication". (Anonymous).

Constipation?

Kratom is a diuretic. It removes water from your body, so make sure you drink plenty of water. Some people experience some constipation, many people don't. People who have experienced Kratom constipation describes it as giving birth to a log. That is not funny. For some people it helps if they take

1 tablespoon of organic coconut oil a couple times during the week. Coconut oil is healthy. If constipation is a problem it can be solved with over-the-counter stool softener or smooth move tea. A daily coffee break, (described in the detox rebuild chapter), is a good idea and very helpful.

Some people mix it with Miralax in powder form. It both mask the taste and they avoid constipation.

Hair loss?

Some people say they have experienced hair loss after using Kratom for a period of time and think it is a Kratom side effect, many others disagree and say they don't experience any hair loss at all. Hair loss in is often related to stress, hormones, age, giving birth, medication, bad diet, lack of protein, vitamin D, iron, side effects from medication or lack of vitamins in general. I have a healthy diet and have not experienced any hair loss at all.

Both the alkaloids Rhynchophylline and Corynoxeine are calcium channel blockers and both contain < 1% of the total alkaloid content found in the Kratom leaf. Is it a possible explanation to why some people experience hair loss? I am not sure. They don't deplete the body of calcium in a way that people will experience calcium depletion. The body will receive enough calcium when people eat a healthy diet. Using prescription drugs depletes the body of many very valuable vitamins and minerals. More information about this is in the chapter about vitamins.

People experiencing hair loss for whatever reason, have found helpful solutions.

"I was losing hair long before I started Kratom. It is due to my fibromyalgia. One of the side effects." (HS).

"Me too. I have fibro and a bad liver." ER).

"It's hormones. It's happened to me. When it first happened way before I was ever pregnant I was convinced I'd be bald in 6 months...I'm not years later. Try not to stress about it, it seems to make it worse." (TL).

"I believe you can get hair loss from Kratom. But 40 percent of your hair in four and a half months seems like something else to me. I would get it checked out and not just assume it's the Kratom." (SO).

"Moringa works a bit like Kratom but helps with hair growth if you're convinced it's the Kratom, but I doubt it is." (BL).

"I drink a lot of Kratom and my hair is just fine. It's probably something else." (CB).

"I think many of us with hair loss also have autonomous diseases and question if it's Kratom. I had hair loss prior to it with my condition." (MN).

"Hormones (including thyroid) as well as not enough protein or animal fat. I have been dealing with it too. Rosemary, and rosemary oil on your scalp can help also. (LF).

"Moringa and Calcium. It works. Biotin didn't help a bit. It has something to do with the calcium factor. I have new hair growing in now." (DB).

"Does that really happen? I've been taking Kratom for almost 6 years and I've never had a problem." (SM).

"Yes, and a lot of people were on other meds that cause hair loss before they started Kratom so it could be the preexisting condition, the meds, etc." (CK).

"Shilajit and moringa will fix this." (JL).

"Same thing happened to me, I had also gone vegan as well. I added in calcium and a few other vitamins and as much as I disliked it, I started making myself eat fish once a week. My hair loss immediately stopped and now it's growing back. My thyroid level was also off." (KD).

"I've noticed people have been talking about this side effect. My hair grows like crazy." (MF).

Moringa is used by many people in the Kratom community. Moringa is power-packed with protein, vitamins, minerals and essential amino acids.

CHAPTER NINE

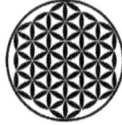

THE KRATOM STRAINS AND VEINS

On the following pages, I will first introduce Kratom in general for people who have chronic disabilities or disorders which force them to take prescription medication, and who wants to use Kratom in a responsible way and thereby reduce their use of prescription medication, which often has many serious side-effects. Then I will go more in depth and reflect upon how to successfully wean off Opiates, street drug, and prescription medication. If you are planning to wean off an addiction and intend to use Kratom for a temporary period of time, then take your time to read everything in this book, because it has valuable information and you want that information. Prepare yourself for a successful lifestyle change.

There are 3 main strains of Kratom. Red, Green, and White.

Red strain: Reduces pain, withdrawal symptoms, and cravings. For some people it is uplifting. It can be either sedating or energizing depending on the vein.

Green strain: Reduces cravings, depression, anxiety, and panic attacks. Elevates mood and increases mental focus. It can be either calming or energizing, depending on the vein.

White strain: Reduces pain and depression. This strain is especially known for its energizing and uplifting qualities. For some people, the white strain has a calming effect, it is often used by people diagnosed with ADHD and ADD. People prone to anxiety might want to mix the white strain with other strains. Using the white strain on its own can give some people jitters and may increase anxiety

Yellow: Typically, white vein leaf which has been sun-dried on the trees.

Gold: Typically, red vein leaf which has been sun-dried on the trees.

> *"Kratom is rather amazing…Comes VERY close to the pain-killing strength of Oxycodone. I have found, that one must find the right dose and the right strain, AND the right vendor. There are strains that have virtually no effect on my pain. The fast-acting veins, like Maeng Da work best for me, adjusting to the correct dose and not taking doses too frequently are key. Taking too much does make one nauseous. "But, if you have not shopped around and experimented with strains then one cannot judge whether Kratom can work for you. Kind of like complimentary pain therapies…if one hasn't tried a variety of them and given them sufficient time and consistent practice one cannot say they don't work. But, find the right type of Kratom and you can forget about*

worrying about access to Opioids...and the energy boost is an added bonus". (F).

"Red Thai and Red MD are generally considered to be the two most energetic red strains of Kratom. For night time, I recommend Red Horn, Red Borneo, or Red Bentuangie. These should still minimize your withdrawal symptoms, but also are relaxing and may help you sleep". (SB).

Kratom is a diuretic and can dehydrate you if you don't drink enough water. Drink plenty of water during the day. Dehydration in general, regardless of Kratom, can give headaches or constipation. Always make sure you stay hydrated.

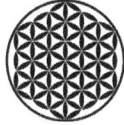

CHAPTER TEN

EXAMPLES OF DIFFERENT KRATOM STRAINS AND VEINS

T he name for a specific Kratom vein does not mean that it is from that specific area, ie. Red Sumatra. Kratom plants are grown in a variety of places in Asia, but the name indicates what kind of qualities are related to the plant. Many vendors sell blends or have renamed Kratom veins. From my personal experience I value the primary strains and veins, then if I want to mix anything together I can do that myself.

These are just a variety of examples of general Kratom qualities so results may vary. It is not intended to diagnose, cure or treat any disease.

- **RED BANJAR** —Strong red sedating very great for relaxing and pain.

- **RED BALI** —Mild, sense of well-being not sedating.

- **RED MAENG DA** —Energetic red great pain relieve, gives energy, and stamina.

- **RED VEIN** —A typical red mild yet effective.

- **RED JONGKONG** —A strong red quick onset can be sedating.

- **SUPER RED MD** —Quick onset, very strong pain relieving and sedating.

- **RED BORNEO** —Deep relaxation, strong, great for sleep.

- **RED HULU** —Good for sleep.

- **RED KALI** —Energetic red.

- **RED HORN** —Great for sleep, deep relaxation and strong pain.

- **RED BALI BLISS** —Quick onset, deeply relaxing.

- **BENTUANGUIE** —Good for sleep and relaxation.

- **RED SUMATRA** —Not sedating, sense of happiness, smooth energy then relaxed.

- **RED VIETNAM** —Very similar to Red Sumatra but more sedating qualities.

- **RED THAI** —Energetic to most, great for pain, energy or sedation based on dosage.

- **RED GOLD** —Mild sense of happiness and well-being. Not sedating.

- **GOLD BANJAR** —Powerful and strong extreme relaxation.

- **GREEN BANJAR** —Strong mildly energetic and enhancing focus.

- **GREEN MEANG DA** —Very strong energetic at lower dose, sedating at higher.

- **GREEN VEIN** —Mildly energetic with an amazing mood boost.

- **GREEN JONGKONG** —Strong focus "get stuff done" strain.

- **GREEN MALAY** —Relaxing, mood boost.

- **GREEN ELEPHANT** —Excellent mood boost, with energy.

- **GREEN THAI** —Great focus.

- **GREEN BALI** —Relaxing, and like typical Bali.

- **SUPER GREEN INDO** —Energetic and great mood boost.

- **SUPER GREEN** —Energetic and great mood boost.

- **GREEN HULU** Relaxing, very strong, slightly sedating, great mood boost, good for anxiety.

- **GREEN BORNEO** —Strong relaxing sedating to some, good for anxiety.

- **WHITE BANJO** —Strong very energetic smooth energy and mood boost.

- **WHITE MD** —Smooth energy, mood boost.

- **WHITE HULU** —Strong energy.

- **WHITE BALI** —Smooth energy.

- **WHITE KALI** —Smooth energy and great mood boost.

- **WHITE JONGKONG** —Mild energy yet relaxed.

- **WHITE THAI** —Energetic.

- **YELLOW MAENG DA** —Deep relaxation, good for anxiety as well.

- **YELLOW JONGKONG** —Strong amazing mood boost and relaxation, yet energetic not sedating.

- **SUPER YELLOW INDO** —Very energetic.

- **HULU KAPUAS** —Mild calming sense of well-being without sedation.

- **BROWN** —Energetic to some, sedating to others. Comfortable relaxation.

At FlowerOfLife808.com You can find high quality organic natural Kratom leaf powder without any additives, tested for salmonella, mold and E-coli etc.

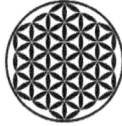

CHAPTER ELEVEN

HOW TO DOSE

"Kratom users can expect to experience full effects in about 30 to 60 minutes after ingestion, although onset can be noticeable after 10-20 minutes. The effects of Kratom typically lasts 5-7 hours with the strongest effect after 2-4 hours after ingestion." (Dr. Henningfield 2016).

This information is intended to help you explore, record, adjust your Kratom intake so it works for you in the most positive way. It is essential that you take responsibility for your own success with Kratom by recording your dosage and outcomes. This would be you writing in a dedicated structured journal, your own LOG BOOK with dosages and reactions recorded each time you ingest Kratom until you know what works for you. This way you can adjust your intake for maximum success.

DOSAGE

Be aware of how you dose and with what you dose. Measure carefully and record doses. I use a measuring spoon set; this way I always measure the right amount. Dosage is especially important for those who search for a specific pain-reducing effect. If the dose is too low there will not be enough pain reducing effect. If the dose is way too high, people will experience "wobbles" or nausea and vomiting. It is not possible to overdose on Kratom and have a fatal outcome. Worst-case scenario is nausea and vomiting while you have to rest for a period of time. (It is my personal experience that Kratom usually takes about 20 minutes to take effect. I mix Kratom with a liquid and drink it.)

Some people take Kratom on an empty stomach, for quick release and medical benefits. Other people choose to take Kratom after food or with food because on an empty stomach it can give them nausea. It will then take longer to activate the Kratom. It is up to the individual person.

Note: The first 2-3 times I tried Kratom I noticed a minor tingling in my hands and a short period with heartbeat and sweating before I felt relaxed. Nothing scary, I just noticed it and assumed it was my body re-adjusting to first time experience of ingesting something new my body wasn't used to. It is a normal first-time reaction for some when using Kratom.

Dosage by teaspoon:

½ —1 teaspoon	Mild
1—2 teaspoons	Medium
2—3 ½ teaspoons	High

Dosage by grams:

1-2 grams	Mild
2—4 ½ grams	Medium
4 ½ —8 grams	High

ALWAYS START LOW when you don't know your tolerance level.

START WITH 1/2 TEASPOON AND WAIT 1/2 HOUR! (Kratom you may have used in the past may be lower quality or strength.) If the desired outcome isn't reached, add another ½ teaspoon and wait. Remember that "less is better." Taking a higher dose than needed might just give "wobbles"(flu-like symptoms), or increase tolerance in general. Some people do not increase intolerance or dosage at all. When it comes to time between dosages, each person is unique and the reason for taking Kratom is different. We all have different metabolism. Likewise, some strains are fast reacting, some are slow reacting. Some strains last longer than others. In general, an appropriate dose usually lasts 4-6 hours. A person weaning off opioids, street drugs or prescription medication will dose differently during withdrawal. (See the chapter about tapering and reducing withdrawal).

"Wobbles" can occur when a person takes too high a dose. It is a side effect of Kratom when taken in a higher dose than current tolerance level. The eyes become wobbly and the sight is unusual. It is difficult to focus at a specific point. It can be followed by headache and nausea. Because it impacts the vision, one should stay away from driving and using machinery or knives. "Wobbles" is unpleasant but temporary. Lie down and rest, or eat and or drink something which will absorb some of the Kratom and also speed up the digestion and help reduce the "wobbles" symptoms.

Use less Kratom next time.

Some strains are more prone to give a "wobbles" effect.

Bali and Green Malaysian can easily give "wobbles" if used over the person's tolerance level while Maeng Da and Thai are much more gentle.

TOLERANCE

Building up a tolerance over time is usually related to people who have chosen to replace prescription medication with Kratom. We can all develop an increased tolerance to almost anything. More food, more sugar, more games, more sex, more cigarettes, more social media, more alcohol, more Oxycodone or whatever is being ingested or used for comfort. High tolerance can happen when a person uses high amounts of Kratom over a prolonged period of time, or when "enhanced products" i.e. a ratio of 10:1—50:1 are used. (1 teaspoon has the same strength as 10 or 50 teaspoons). High tolerance can be reduced significantly or reset by taking a couple of days off once in a while. Some choose to take one or two days off from Kratom during the week. Some take a few days off every couple of weeks. That will keep the tolerance low.

"I do a tolerance reset every 6-8 weeks for 3-4 days. I haven't experienced withdrawal, but I don't take Kratom for Opiate withdrawal, I take it for pain and energy so that may be a factor." (SP).

"Everyone is different, I don't get withdrawals from Kratom, I stopped cold turkey and didn't have any withdrawals. I've been taking around 20-30 g (10-15 tsp) Kratom a day for almost 4 years. I take a 3-5 day break (reset break to avoid SSS, Same Strain Syndrome) every 4-6 weeks. I experience a couple of psychological withdrawal symptoms like anxiety, but NOTHING like Opiate withdrawals. I'd much rather cope with Kratom than Opiates." (NM).

"Switch strains or take a break. I take low dose 3 X a day and it's replaced antidepressants for me. I have taken Kratom for 13 years and have managed to keep a low tolerance." (PR).

(SSS/ Same Strain Syndrome: When a person only uses the same strain and does it very often, it results in a higher dose with lower impact than usual, and can be reduced/eliminated by rotating veins and strains).

Try these habits to avoid SSS tolerance and keep your dosage low:

- One can change the strains during the day i.e. white, green and red.)
- One can change between veins during the day i.e. Red MD (Red Maeng Da), Red Thai and Red Horn.
- One can use a different vein or strain for each day during the week.
- One can use one strain for a week or a month and then change to a different strain.
- One can change vein or strain every couple day.
- One can change strain every other week.
- One can use stem and leaf for a few days. In between strains.

DO NOT DISSOLVE KRATOM FOR INJECTION! It can give you an infection and it will not give any desired or positive outcome. It doesn't work that way and it is a waste of time, energy and money. Kratom works ORALLY.

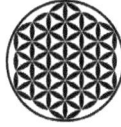

CHAPTER TWELVE

LOGBOOK

B esides the general qualities of the individual veins, (Ex. Green Malay), finding the right strains and veins for you is a personal quest. If you think that only one strain, vein or dose will ease everything you might be disappointed. We all metabolize differently, have different weight, height, different purpose for using Kratom and different ways of ingesting it. One strain might do wonders for one person but not another. Then find the right dosage. It is a good idea to take your time to make a logbook and write down strains, veins, reactions, and doses and learn from that, especially if you have chronic pain and intend to replace prescription medication with Kratom. Even writing a journal can be very beneficial. It is well worth the time.

Having a chronic disease or chronic pain is hell, even more so if many prescription medications are involved, and especially if the prescription medications have serious side effects. Many people have successfully eliminated or reduced prescription medications with Kratom.

There are several Kratom strains and veins. They have common traits which work for many people and then there are some people who experience adverse reactions to Kratom. While the majority will experience the general effects, a small percentage experience the opposite effect. For example, if the strain is energetic they will be relaxed, if the strain is relaxing they might feel energized. People diagnosed with ADHD have, for example, experienced the high energetic white vein to be relaxing.

Some people have tried Kratom and didn't hit their sweet spot the first time, and lacking this knowledge, gave up on finding relief because they thought Kratom didn't work. Find the sweet spot.

For some chronic disease or chronic pain patients it may take some trial and error before they find what exactly works for them individually. Those who investigate, who try and maybe fail a couple of times often end up with success. If they have used a logbook and logged it, they know exactly what strains and veins work for them, how much to take, how often, how to take it, what relief they get, and they now have knowledge of how to make their own specific blends that work wonders for them.

A great way to figure out what works for you is through creating a logbook and log your use.

There are different ways to make a logbook, but for it to be effective, there has to be valuable information.

- ## DATE.
- ## TIME.
- ## AMOUNT.
- ## STRAIN AND VEIN.
- ## HOW IT WAS INGESTED.

Feedback information. (Length of time before reaction, the kind of experiences and reaction, etc.).

Below is an example of my own logbook.

8/21/15. 1:40 p.m. ½ teaspoon. Green vein. Mixed in water. (Strong taste. Very diffuse experience, I can feel something but not really clear enough to indicate what). Need a higher dose.

8/21/15. 2:50 p.m. An additional ¼ teaspoon. Green vein. Mixed in water. (Strong taste. After 20 minutes I started getting very relaxed and tired. I laid down on my bed and relaxed, a stressful thought which under normal circumstances would easily unease me, was easy to redirect with very little emotional interference. If a thought about food popped up (the munchies), it was easy to redirect. I had an overall feeling of well-being and relaxation. It was easy to just witness what was happening without being too emotionally attached. Lasted 4-5 hours. (relaxing, anti-stress, anti-anxiety, overall well-being).

8/21/15. 9:52 p.m. ½ + teaspoon. Red Horn. Mixed in tea with Pau d'Arco, Tulsi, Dandelion, Thyme, Masala Chai and honey. (Strong taste. After 20 minutes, relaxed and resting. It is not hard for me to redirect an emotional thought or to focus on meditation or specific thoughts. No pain after intense physical exercise. (didn't sleep deep or much during the night, interesting since a lot of people experience Red Horn as a sedative, maybe it was because of the late evening exercise or low dose? Try again).

8/22/15. 12.00 p.m. ½+ teaspoon of Green Borneo. Feeling very well, energetic, optimistic and happy. Got plenty of things done.

8/22/15. 10.00 p.m. 1 teaspoon of Red Horn. Very relaxed and slept all night. My favorite night time strain. 1/4 -1/2 teaspoon was too little.

After some trial and possible errors, you will have your logbook and know your strains, veins, and what you can mix together.

"I find that sometimes I get best results by making blends of different strains. If you have a strain that doesn't seem to be working great for you, try mixing it with another strain and you'll often get different or even better effects." (KC).

"I usually mix greens and yellows for day time and reds and yellows for night." (BE).

"I have a jar I called 'leftovers' that has some of every color and different strain in it. It's actually my favorite." (SJ).

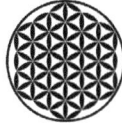

CHAPTER THIRTEEN

WAYS TO INGEST KRATOM

TW means toss and wash. A number of Kratom users prefer this quick method. It usually takes 15-20 minutes to work. Put the Kratom powder in your mouth and wash it down with liquid. Likewise there are even more people who really don't like this method because they have ended up blowing all the powder out or inhaling it. On top of that, the taste can be really bad, like sour green leaf. None of them are fun, at all. It can be pretty painful to inhale it and I don't think it is good for the lungs. Blowing it out is a waste of good Kratom, and for sure you might want to mask the taste. You can always give it a try and quickly figure out if it is something for you or not.

The easiest way is to just mix it with liquid and drink it. You can use any liquid but some are better than others, especially if you want to mask the taste of greens or at best mask the taste of green tea powder.

These are examples of liquids you can mix with Kratom. Chocolate almond milk, apple sauce, coffee, pink grape juice, yoghurt, chocolate milk, elderberry juice, coffee creamer, there are many possibilities. Over time you will find the one the suits you best. I myself use a little mason jar glass container with a plastic lid. Add the desired amount of Kratom, add the liquid, shake it and drink it.

> *"Dose in bottom of glass or plastic bottle you can shake. Add lemon juice (potentiator), and some warm water (2-3 oz). Shake it. Add orange juice or grapefruit juice. Shake, shake, shake. Let it rest for 5-10 minutes and then drink it. (the warm water dissolves the powder, it doesn't even taste bad either." (JW).*

Lemon balls: Mix with very little lemon juice and make a dough. Roll the dough for easier cutting dosage or roll pills and put them in the refrigerator or the freezer.

Honey balls: Mix with very little honey and make a dough. Roll the dough for easier cutting dosage or roll pills. If the dough is rolled in powdered sugar it will be less sticky. Put them in the refrigerator or the freezer.

KRATOM TEA RECIPE

Making tea for just one dose of Kratom is both time and energy consuming. You can do it but ask yourself if it is worth doing that when you can make almost a gallon at the same time as one dose.

Kratom tea: 50 grams Kratom per gallon. Cinnamon, 1-2 oranges and a pinch of salt to reduce the bitterness, sweet and spicy tea bags as you prefer.

Simmer for 25-30 minutes on low heat. Don't boil it. Strain it if needed. Be aware that when you boil or strain the tea you may also boil or strain away some of the beneficial Kratom alkaloids.

You can add sugar or honey to sweeten the tea.

Kratom tea can be stored in mason jars in the refrigerator for around 5 days.

CAPSULES

Buying pre-made capsules with Kratom is often pretty expensive and can contain additives. It is cheaper to buy Kratom powder and make capsules yourself but keep in mind that you have to take quite a lot of capsules when you take a dose. You can buy a capsule filling device and veggie capsules on Amazon.

Some people prefer capsules because they don't like the taste of Kratom. When capsules are used it takes a longer time before there is an effect. It is good idea to poke holes in the capsule with a needle for a faster response.

Size 00 capsule = 0.5 g = ¼ teaspoon.

Size 000 capsule = 0.8 g = ¾ teaspoon.

STORAGE

Mason jars, tightly closed plastic bags, dark containers. If Kratom is stored in a cool, dark place it can keep the potency for up to 2 years or more. Any storage in the refrigerator or freezer has to be sealed really tight. You don't want any moisture in your Kratom. Freezing Kratom will stop the decomposition.

KRATOM POTENTIATORS

There are different ways to enhance the qualities of Kratom and thereby lower the dose, often as much as half of what a person would normally take. Only 1 potentiator is needed per dose. The potentiator slows down the body's metabolism, and therefore also slows down the enzymes which break down the Kratom alkaloids. It will make the dose stronger and last longer. Pay attention to how much you dose when you use a potentiator; use less than you usually use.

Common potentiators include: Lemon juice, orange juice, grapefruit juice, Emergen—C, starfruit juice, watercress, apple cider vinegar, tonic water, chamomile tea, magnesium, turmeric powder, cayenne pepper powder, black pepper powder, ginger root ground.

Turmeric and pepper needs a fatty oil like coconut oil to be activated as a potentiator. Not a bad idea since coconut oil is a great health supplement and will help with bathroom visits.

For maximum results, many people have good experience with taking the ground potentiators 20—30 minutes before their Kratom dose. Yet again, we are all different individual beings and we metabolize differently.

You can, for example, mix turmeric, finely ground pepper and ground ginger with coconut oil, drink it and then take Kratom dose.

Some people have reduced their Kratom dosage by freezing their Kratom mixed with lemon juice.

> *"I used to mix my Kratom in lemon juice and wait 5 minutes or more before using. Longer time didn't seem to make a difference. So, for freezing I used roughly 3 times the lemon juice by volume to Kratom powder. I have a tiny little plastic container that is perfect for this. Freezing it until red rings appear. I have been able to cut my dose in half from 1 tablespoon to ½ a tablespoon, and instead of having to dose every 3 1/4 hours to 4, now I'm only dosing every 6 hours. Whatever seems to happen in the freezing process seems to be effective. It also doesn't seem as nearly as bitter after being frozen." (RB).*

> *"I just mix a quarter cup of lemon juice, a half cup of water and 8g of my favorite Kratom. I freeze it for 5 hours (see the red ring), thaw it and drink.... It is different.... Not a bad thing. Try it". (TH).*

KRATOM TIPS

*The more severe the nerve damage or current high-level opiate use, the longer it can take to find the right strain and the right dosage. If the receptors are blocked the full Kratom benefits and potential may not be experienced immediately. Some people have gone directly from opioids to Kratom with no problems. Take the time to investigate the different strains and veins by using your logbook notes.

Some veins become sedative when taken in high dosage.

*Strains and veins can vary in potency depending on different factors. Time of the year it is harvested, where it was planted, sun, weather and soil conditions, how old the powder is, etc.

WHAT DID KRATOM DO FOR ME?

After a couple of intense and stressful years my sleep was affected. Some days I slept as little as a couple hours and I noticed that I started to become depressed and my diet became unhealthy. I researched and tried to find a natural way to increase my sleep, then I found Kratom and discovered its magnificent benefits. It ended up with a lifestyle change.

Due to lack of information I read somewhere that all red strains are sedative, so I ordered Red Maeng Da. Which turned out to be a mistake since Red maeng Da is energetic. 3 evenings in a row I took it at bedtime and ended up with no sleep at all. I found out that some red strains are sedative and others are energizing. Then I ordered Red Horn, a sedative strain and that was what I needed.

1 to 1 ½ teaspoon at night time was what helped me to relax and sleep much better.

During daytime I often take 1 to 1 ½ teaspoon of energetic super green or green jong kong. The energy and the uplifting and positive effect was what gave me energy to go to the gym and exercise. I have never experienced a rise in tolerance; neither have I experienced any withdrawal symptoms from Kratom. I usually do a 2-day reset during the week and often I forget to take the Kratom at evening time or during the day.

I decided to do a natural rebalancing of my dopamine, serotonin and endorphin levels by juicing vegetables, fruit, a varied diet and exercise. It works miracles. I get my sleep and I wake up early focused and energetic. I feel much more in balance physically, mentally and emotionally.

I start every morning with Raw B complex a high potency whole food complex formula, Milk Thistle, DLPA, 32 ounces of green juice or a Purium (described later) shake to replenish my body with vitamins and minerals and I do a coffee break (explained in the health chapter), to detox my body of any toxins. Some hours later I take the green strain and I am ready to exercise.

I have now lost 35 pounds, I am not depressed, I am healthy, and I love my lifestyle. A very welcome side effect for me personally, I lost all cravings for sugar and lost interest in alcohol. Kratom can help reduce withdrawal symptoms and cravings for alcohol for light and medium alcohol addictions.

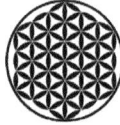

CHAPTER FOURTEEN

DRUG WITHDRAWAL SYMPTOMS

Below I will describe ordinary and common withdrawal symptoms which happen during an initial wean off period of around 7-14 days, sometimes less, sometimes more. This is essential to understand why so many people keep using prescription medication or drugs over and over again. Weaning off without the proper support like Kratom, DPLA, healthy diet and exercise is basically 7-14 days of hell physically, psychologically and emotionally.

> *"I use heroin/Fentanyl very heavily, and the withdrawals were absolute torture." (HD).*

> *"Yesterday was my FIRST DAY CLEAN... I WANNA CONTINUE BUT WITHDRAWAL SYMPTOMS AND CRAVINGS ARE OVERWHELMING! DON'T KNOW HOW TO HANDLE IT." (PS).*

Clinical expert says; "People continue to take drugs to avoid withdrawal symptoms." Instead of running away from Gray Death (10,000 times stronger than Morphine), they run towards it because they feel it is strong enough to help them not get sick. (USA Today May 24th. 2017).

> *"I'm clean for 5 months, but that's a crazy lifestyle. I used to steal, lie, all kinds of crazy shit. Life is so much better now."* (PM).

> *"People hustle, beg, borrow and steal just to keep the buzz rolling and eventually just to keep the withdrawal away."* (CT).

> *"I had played with Lortabs in the past, but this time it was more than play. Started taking about 30 to 40 mg a day. Toward the end it was nothing to take 100 to 150 mg daily. I did not have a script. The 10 mg tab cost seven dollars. Do the math. I maxed out my credit cards and got four different loans and that doesn't include borrowing money from coworkers and friends. Toward the end the only reason I was taking them was to avoid withdrawal. Today is 17 days clean and day 2 without Kratom. It did serve its purpose."* (MM).

Active users will do whatever they can to not experience the withdrawal symptoms (any kind of crime, prostitution, lies, etc.), or when withdrawals start to arrive, active users go into panic and will do whatever it takes to avoid them, including taking whatever other drug, no matter what drug, simply to avoid the incoming withdrawal symptoms.

WHAT ARE THE GENERAL DRUG WITHDRAWAL SYMPTOMS?

Vomiting, nausea, diarrhea, insomnia, restless legs, shaking, cramps, cold chills, nightmares, sweating, anxiety, panic attacks, depression, loss of appetite, fatigue, delusions, brain fog, seizures. (draxe.com 2016, et al.).

> *"For an addict in active addiction there is one goal on their mind every single morning. To NOT be sick." (TT).*

> *"I stayed on Methadone two years due to the fact that I was deathly afraid of the withdrawals." (CS).*

> *"I didn't know about Kratom like this back then. For 10 straight days, I crawled from my bed to the toilet, sweat buckets 24/7, wanted to cut my legs off and just in general thought I was dying. I remember how big a shock to the body it is when you are physically and physiologically dependent on this level. (Nausea, diarrhea and restless legs are normal withdrawal symptoms). Kratom just makes it easier." (SE).*

Experiencing these withdrawals is often referred to as going "cold turkey", (quitting without first tapering down and without help from prescription medications or Kratom). Very few people are able to go through this insane process without help. It is so intense that people think they are dying. Nobody wants to be going through a week or two of hell like this, thinking they are dying. Cramping in insane pain on the floor while vomiting, pooping and peeing all over at the same time. Some active users, when weaning off, choose to be held in a very expensive induced medical coma for a period of time because withdrawal symptoms are so insane. Withdrawal symptoms are the reason why many users end up on "maintenance" drugs like Methadone, Suboxone, Subutex, etc. for years or the rest of their life, which by the way, have the same or worse withdrawal symptoms if the maintenance drug is not taken as prescribed.

According to feedback, many former users have been able to wean off various drugs with very little to no withdrawal symptoms when using Kratom. In most cases Kratom can reduce the above described withdrawal symptoms by up to 75-90%. At this level, withdrawal symptoms become manageable. It can still be somewhat unpleasant, but absolutely nothing compared to 7-14 days of hell. Some former users have reported having no withdrawal symptoms at all.

Take your time to read the information below:

"Well today is day 3 of Kratom and day 2 of no pain pills.... all I have to say is I'm loving this stuff!!!! I can feel the withdrawals a little but with this I can actually function... thank god I decided to give it a try. Seriously I'd be going crazy right now on day 2 no meds..." (DC).

"I stopped taking Opiates and started taking Kratom, and had no withdrawal symptoms. I was on Opiates for 20+ years on very high doses. (I used red strains)". (PD).

"I had tried to quit painkillers 100 times. I would end up giving up because the withdrawal was so bad. I've been clean 25 days today, with Kratom. I wouldn't believe it if I wasn't living it. It is amazing." (BG).

"I used Red Bali to kick 120 Mg Roxycodone per day, with almost no withdrawals at all." (MS).

"I used opiates for 14 years for pain and they just gave me more and more, but no more thanks to KRATOM. It saved me. No withdrawal and it helps a lot for the pain. (MK)."

"I have Muscular Dystrophy and was on Vyvanse (similar to Adderall) and decided I wanted to quit. Every other time I quit I had severe withdrawals. This time I used Kratom for withdrawals and didn't experience any withdrawals. (CU)."

"I used Kratom in July 2016 to get off methadone prescribed for pain. I used it consistently for 3 months, several doses a day and had zero withdrawal. Opiate free for over a year. Good luck! You are doing great. Subs and Bups are the devil." (GA).

"I never experienced withdrawals when detoxing with Kratom. Kratom helps so much." (LM).

"I have been off Suboxone for 2 weeks, thanks to Kratom. Almost zero withdrawals." (JD).

"I'm on day 8 after switching from Morphine to Kratom. I tapered down morphine and then when I got Kratom I switched over. Almost zero withdrawal symptoms. I have multiple chronic pain conditions and finding the right strain for the right pain is proving to be the only tricky part so far. For withdrawals it was perfect." (SH).

"Kratom saved my life. Full blown addiction to Crystal Meth and Opiates and I weaned off both with Kratom, with little to no withdrawal symptoms." (KK).

"It's been 3 weeks since I started detoxing off Methadone and today I'm feeling great. My energy and sense of happiness is coming back. Thanks to Kratom, Kratom helped me off of the hardest drugs out there. Methadone withdrawals are the worst. I'm so glad I beat it without having to go through the horror. (AP).

"I was an IV heroin user. I kicked it cold turkey with Kratom, it saved my life. I'm clean almost 80 days. It helped with all my withdrawals." (RB).

"My boy overdosed and died in front of me, I stopped IV heroin cold turkey. I took Kratom to help with the withdrawals and I haven't looked back since. The worst is only 3 days!" (BR).

Kratom might not reduce withdrawals 100% for everyone, but there is no doubt that it works for the majority of people, maybe as high as 90% of people. Later I will discuss DLPA. DLPA will reduce withdrawals and cravings even more.

Remember that this is your life's mission. This is about saving your life, nothing less and it is not only about you, but children, siblings, parents, uncles, aunties, cousins, grandparents, good friends, and your dog, cat, bird or pet rat, pet spider or pet flower. They all want you back. Prepare yourself the best you can so you can have success.

Weaning off with Kratom (and the later introduced DLPA) makes most people able to still function in their daily life and take care of family, work and study during the withdrawal process.

Often when the 1-2 week wean-off period is over, former users get to really experience what Kratom is. Keep in mind that Opioids etc., block the synapses in the brain and have a half-life period of time where Kratom cannot be experienced in its full potential. This is usually when "now former" opioid and street drug users start to taper down various other medications, prescribed or not, because of side effects related to the original drug use.

PAWS. POST-ACUTE WITHDRAWAL SYMPTOMS

After the initial wean off period of 1-2 weeks with withdrawals, people start to get much better, it also starts a longer period with frequent and temporary PAWS (Post-Acute Withdrawal Symptoms), for most former users. These can be temporary symptoms like cravings, anxiety, depression, fatigue, mood swings, panic attack, insomnia etc. It can be very unpleasant but is temporary. Over time there will be longer gaps between the symptoms, and the time during the symptoms will be shorter. PAWS (Post-Acute Withdrawal Symptoms) are likely to pop up once in a while and can last a couple of days, during the following months or longer. No matter what, stay strong and things will be better. Having Kratom, DLPA and later mentioned specific over-the-counter supplements on hand will most likely save your day and prevent you from going back to drugs. PAWS are temporary and usually take less than a couple of days.

Some former users continue to keep red Kratom on hand for PAWS, then use the green Kratom strains for a couple of months because these are pain killing, give energy, reducing cravings, reducing anxiety, reducing depression and are mood enhancing. The white strain is often mixed in because it is energizing.

After the initial withdrawals, the brain is now going to rebalance dopamine, and endorphins etc. again. Furthermore, the body starts a natural detox and healing process. Some PAWS are most likely healing reactions of the body/brain releasing toxins. You can actively take part in the process and work with the healing process and see the PAWS as a confirmation that your body is healing. Change something seemingly negative to something positive. The more time and energy you invest in this process, the more control you have, and the faster you will heal and come through to the other side, stronger than you have ever felt. **You got this!**

The most important thing you can ever invest in is your health!

During this process, you might need help or support from rehab groups, FB groups, a therapist or a Cognitive Behavioral Psychologist. This way you have like-minded people or a professional to talk with about the former use/abuse, and to heal whatever physical, mental or emotional wounds there might be. Especially if your use was ignited by or related to sexual abuse, violence, addicted parents, the death of family member or a close friend, etc. There are other things you can do for yourself, which will support you and help rebuild you in the chapter "How I coped with anxiety, panic attacks and depression without using pharmaceutical drugs".

CHANGING BAD HABITS TO GOOD HABITS

Habits can-be difficult to break. What if you can replace a bad habit with a good habit and become addicted to good habits? Yes, it is possible.

The MKE (The Master Key Experience is based on the book "The Master Key" written by Charles F. Haanel). The MKE has recently been of tremendous value for me and thousands of other people. I have replaced bad habits with new good habits.

I can highly recommend it to support your decision to wean off an addiction or for any business project you want success in. MKE offers FREE SCHOLARSHIPS paid forward by previous members. It is free to sign up and months later you decide if you want to pay for a scholarship forward for someone else. MKE has certified guides and their tools and techniques to reach goals are amazing.

I easily implemented positive and uplifting thoughts, juicing every day and exercising every day. These three components will help you tremendously in your detox and rebuilding process. I have detoxed and rejuvenated my physical and mental being. I went from 201.5 pounds to 169.5 pounds. I lost 32+ pounds and am now strong and healthy. Instead of going to bed at 2-3 o'clock in the morning I now go to bed around 11 p.m. and wake up at sunrise. I still juice and exercise daily and I reach my goals. Everything I do benefits me and my family.

Go to masterkeyexperience.com to get a free scholarship.

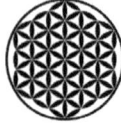

CHAPTER FIFTEEN

WHAT TO DO WHEN YOU WANT TO WEAN

IMPORTANT: People diagnosed with severe depression (endogenous/clinical depression) should be under medical and psychological supervision and NOT just wean off their medication. For people diagnosed with endogenous/ clinical depression, psychiatric medication and continuous evaluation are important and lifesaving. Consult with your medical provider before doing anything.

P eople with situational depression related to a specific incident should keep in mind that situational depression is temporary and will be healed over time.

Know that you can do it. Anyone motivated to stop using can stop and be successful. For some people it is easier than expected, for others it is a longer process. Remember the suffering is temporary. When you are done with drugs you will be healthier, stronger and happier than before. Many people have used Kratom to come off drugs by themselves. Maybe they were successful because they got control over their situation and did it in their own environment which gave them time for physical and psychological adjustments.

When you decide to wean off an addiction to opioids, street drugs or prescription medication and want to increase your success, there are important things you want to take into consideration:

1. Plan it in advance. Prepare, prepare, prepare. Read this manual to the end. Make sure that you have enough Kratom and supplements etc. so you don't run out. Especially read the chapter on how to cope with anxiety, panic attacks and depression without using pharmaceuticals, there may be some good suggestions you can use. Kratom can reduce or eliminate cravings and withdrawal symptoms and most anxiety and depressive thoughts but it is good to know how to cope with it anyway. Most people still experience PAWS (Post-Acute Withdrawal Symptoms) after the initial withdrawal period.

2. Your list of friends. Your dealer is not your friend. You've got to admit this right away. In your dealer's eyes, you are just a cash cow. The more you spend on drugs the happier your dealer gets, and your dealer doesn't really care what you get and if you die…. He doesn't care about your family either. The same with your "drug-using friends;" those who use drugs often or every day, usually only have one thing in common:

drugs…. They will try to get you hooked on drugs again. It will make them feel better that they are not the only ones using drugs. You will have to replace them with friends who care for you and like you for who you are.

You need to disconnect 100% from your dealer or "friends" because they will try to contact you to push you into drug use again…….

3. Get a new phone number. You need to erase as many phone numbers as possible to dealers and "friends", it is absolutely best if you get a new phone number and keep it clean from anything which can drag you back into using drugs.

4. Move away. Sometimes people will have to move away and start a new life, which is basically what sometimes happens when people wean off a drug. They start a new life.

"My Suboxone addiction was a physical addiction due to the chemicals that made me physically dependent after taking the drug for a period of time. (Kratom saved my ass from that. Drugs like meth and cocaine used to be mentally addictive for me. Since I have been taking Kratom and changed my people, places and things, and my ways of thinking, I don't feel compelled to waste my time with that shit anymore." (JD).

You don't want to relapse into drugs again because it may cost you your life.

TAPERING

Tapering is gradually reducing your dose, it is distributing withdrawal symptoms over a longer period of time and minimizing the discomfort experienced when weaning off. A gradual and sufficiently slow, step by step stop from drugs will give the body's natural systems the ability to regain control of normal functions again. Juicing, detoxing and exercising will speed up the healing process and are perfectly good habits to implement in your lifestyle change. See the suggestions on how to naturally cope with anxiety, panic attacks and depression which are described later.

For some drugs, such as benzodiazepines and alcohol if used heavily and over a long period of time, it can be very important to taper because they can cause life-threatening seizures and be extremely unpleasant to stop using abruptly. The higher the dose the more important it is to taper. Tapering will drastically increase the success of fully quitting. Because all drugs in general have a different half-life (the time it takes for the drug to reduce by 50%), it is a good idea to know what the specific half-life is. The longer the half-life, the longer it will take before the initial withdrawal symptoms begin.

> *"I was taking 40mg of Dilaudid several times a day... You can do this. I don't know how I'm alive, but I promise Kratom will help. I lowered to 12mg 6x a day over 2 months then went with Kratom." (LM).*

> *"I was taking almost ten 50mg Tramadol a day for 8 months. I tapered and then quit. I used Kratom for withdrawals and*

I definitely suffered but I survived and was even functional and active (day 3 and 4 withdrawals were hell). Kratom made it tolerable." (BK).

"I did it after 8+ years on morphine with the help of Kratom and Cannabis. Just make sure you taper, that makes it much easier". (MF).

Some people successfully use Kratom by gradually replacing a drug dose with Kratom. While they are weaning off an unwanted drug, some people fully stop using the drug and only use Kratom during the initial withdrawal symptom period of a couple of weeks. Then they reduce the use of Kratom to fully stop using Kratom and only have it on hand, in case PAWS happens later. Remember that PAWS are temporary and can be reduced or eliminated with Kratom, exercise, a healthy diet, and coping strategies.

TAPERING BENZODIAZEPINES

(Valium, Xanax, Ativan, Librium, Klonopin, etc.).

Benzodiazepines were originally intended to be used for a very short period of time and related to traumatic experiences or as sedatives during surgery. Today they are generally used in the treatment of anxiety, panic disorders, insomnia and depression and are heavily used for recreational purposes. They are tolerance-building and over time they can be very dangerous. People have died from overdose. Benzodiazepine withdrawals can take a long time and if you use Benzodiazepines for too long, you can begin to get what's called paradoxical effects. That is when the drug starts causing the symptoms they were intended to reduce.

Do not just stop Benzodiazepines, you can get life threatening seizures, heart palpitations, audio and visual hallucinations. Taper down.

The general guideline is tapering/reduce the use by 10% or less every 2-4 week. If in doubt or in need of support, contact your medical provider for a more detailed tapering schedule.

"Day 5 with no pain pills, no Percocet and no Xanax and I feel great. Kratom might save my life after all. I was skeptical and it took some work to find the dose that worked. My kids deserve to have a happy and healthy mom." (LM).

"It's 20 months I'm off Xanax, pain pills and alcohol. I feel so much better now." (KJ).

"I just weaned myself off Oxycodone and Diazepam." (KH).

"I quit all pain meds and Xanax with the help of Kratom" (JL).

"Kratom saved my life from 6 years of Oxycontin, Tramadol, and Valium. I thought I could never live without the next pill. Now I'm not slave to the next pill anymore." (KT).

"I have Borderline personality disorder and have come off all my meds and feel better than I have in a long time. I still have anxiety at times but the Kratom has helped manage that as well as depression and my mind has been calmer. I

haven't had any psychosis. I told my therapist about it and she was all for it and has even seen a difference in me. (AG).

"I have severe bipolar II. I've been on dozens of meds. Literally everything one could think of and it barely controlled it. I tried Kratom for chronic pain and discovered it controls the bipolar better than any med. Fast forward a year... I take no psych meds at all. This may not be the case for everyone but for me Kratom was a godsend." (AH).

"I suffer from bipolar disorder borderline personality major depressive disorder anxiety and panic attacks Kratom has replaced all my meds." (SJ).

"I was on 7 psych drugs. Stopped them all after I started Kratom. I have bipolar as well. With a few other diagnoses. Lithium. Seroquel. Buspar. Prozac. Vistaril. Trazadone. Gabapentin. I was on all of those." (DG).

TAPERING SSRI

(Selective Serotonin Reuptake Inhibitors). (Prozac, Zoloft, Celexa, Paxil, Lexapro, Luvox, Effexor etc.).

SSRIs are generally used in the treatment of anxiety, panic disorders, depression, OCD (Obsessive compulsive disorder), and are heavily used for recreational purposes. SSRIs can induce suicide, self-destructive thoughts or self-destructive behavior, violent behavior and mania, and can be associated with anxiety, panic attacks, insomnia and hostility.

The report, called "Psychiatric Drugs Create Violence & Suicide: School Shootings & Other Acts of Senseless Violence," provides information on more than 30 studies that link antidepressants, antipsychotics, psychostimulants, mood stabilizers and sedative hypnotics to adverse effects that include hostility, mania, aggression, self-harm, suicide and homicidal thoughts. (https://www.prnewswire.com).

Read the report at: https://www.cchrint.org/pdfs/violence-report.pdf

"Prozac promotes suicide, violence, psychosis, and mayhem." (MD Peter Breggin 2014).

It is usually recommended to taper down over a minimum of 4-6 weeks if SSRIs have been used in maintenance treatment.

If in doubt or in need of support, contact your medical provider for a more detailed tapering schedule.

"I tapered off the antidepressants while taking Kratom. Pristiq and Prozac." (HC).

"I use half or a whole teaspoon of Green Malay for my severe anxiety and clinical depression. Works great." (BB).

"I have been clean some time now. I choose Kratom as a replacement for my antidepressants and anxiety meds, because before I was self-medicating with Opioids, etc. Now, I want to make it clear that Kratom has taken away any and all cravings for Opioids and anything else." (SS).

"I was alone in trying Kratom, but it was the best decision I could have made. I was on massive amounts of Norco, anxiety meds, sleeping pills and antidepressants. Now, the only thing I take is thyroid med." (LL).

"My chronic condition has totally settled down. Awesome natural pain relief, energy for my kids, no more anxiety or depression, chronic insomnia is gone. The need for alcohol or toxification of any sort goes away. An overall sense of feeling good. Kratom is a Godsend." (TR).

"I'm ten days free of Pristiq because of Kratom, I've had little to no physical withdrawals. In the past, I've tapered my dose and tried to quit them, and the brain fog, fatigue, and dizziness had me going back." (DE).

"Me and my husband will be clean 2 years on New Year's and it's all thanks to Kratom! I also quit my Prozac and Ambien at the same time. No issues, no relapse!" (SF).

"Kratom has replaced my painkillers and is helping me wean off antidepressants. It is a miracle plant." (ML).

"I have chronic depression and anxiety. Kratom works better than any antidepressant I've ever taken, because it doesn't take you up so high and let you crash into a suicidal darkness." (CK).

TAPERING OPIOIDS

(Oxycodone, heroin, Morphine, Methadone, Suboxone, Fentanyl, Norco, Percocet, Vicodin, Buprenorphine, Demerol, etc.).

Opioids were originally intended to be used only by terminally ill people in severe pain and in the end stages of cancer. In recent years Opioids have been used as ordinary pain medication. Opioids (synthetic, and semi-synthetic opiates) are often used as maintenance medication for people who wean off heroin or for pain.

If you have used high doses for a long period of time it is recommended to taper down before you stop.

Slow tapering: 5-20% reduction each month.

Fast tapering: 10-20% reduction each week.

If in doubt or in need of support, contact your medical provider for a more detailed tapering schedule.

> *"Before I found it I was strung out for 4 years on opiates and injecting heroin. First week taking Kratom with withdrawals I could eat, sleep and act normal. After 4 months of Kratom I've been weaning off, now I'm on month 6 and I only take Kratom a few times a week when I feel urges or severe anxiety and depression." (HK).*

> *"I did 10 Percocets a day (just getting high). I eventually found Kratom and was able to kick Percs. Haven't really touched synthetic Opioids since then." (WD).*

"35 days clean from 6 years opiate addiction, my husband showed up with Kratom and I never looked back."

"We both have many medical problems and Kratom has saved our lives." (DD).

"I'm 10 days away from being 1 year clean from 11 years opiate addiction. Opiates ruined my life but I never gave up, and now my life is better than ever. Don't give up. Kratom saved my life, it will save yours too."

"Smoker, drinker, Opioid addict. Now I'm free of all three. I have energy, a positive outlook and I'm mentally healthy." (AJ).

"Today is my 17th month anniversary of finding Kratom and getting off opiates." (MC).

"Freedom from 19 meds, including ALL OPIATES". (DE).

"My boyfriend used red and green strains to wean off Suboxone and it worked wonders." (AW).

"I'm 14 days off Suboxone and my first batch of Kratom worked wonders."

"Just came off Suboxone with the help of Kratom." (PV).

"I used Kratom to get off Suboxone, I started with a red then mixed it with a green, then red/white. Now mostly green/white mix." (MT).

"Kratom practically saved my life, not only do I have depression and anxiety, I have a dozen chronic pain issues.

Because of the pain, I was addicted to opiates for a very long time. Since finding Kratom a little more than a year ago, I have been sober, and my health has improved. I also helped a family member, also with addiction and chronic pain, by recommending Kratom, and am happy to say, she also has been in recovery since beginning Kratom." (S).

TAPERING OFF AEDS (ANTIEPILEPTIC DRUGS) AND ANTICONVULSANTS

(Gabapentin, Lyrica, Neurontin, Clonazepam, Topomax, Horizant, Lamictal, Tegretol, and anti-Parkinsonians).

These drugs are often used for patients suffering from seizures, chronic pain, and neuropathic pain, epilepsy as well as many other neurological and psychiatric conditions. They are widely prescribed for many things and very often they are used to reduce withdrawals from other drugs.

If you have had a difficult time with AEDs and anticonvulsants or suffer from withdrawal symptoms related to them due to high doses, it is important to taper down first. Stopping these medications suddenly can increase seizures.

Slowly taper the medication, you can do a 25% dose reduction, every 2-4 weeks.

If in doubt or in need of support, contact your medical provider for a more detailed tapering schedule.

"Neurontin makes you neurotic...it made me crazy, mean and still don't have much short-term memory...I haven't taken that crap for a year now...it made things worse for me." (AS).

"I took Lyrica which is similar and it made me fall constantly, forget things, and I was so mean." (RS).

"I'm forgetful. I can't talk right half the time. Forget words. Can't comprehend. Basically, I feel like a complete dumbass." (MA).

"They had me on Lyrica, Gabapentin, and Cymbalta at the same time, mediocre pain relief and BIG side effects! Kratom is working way better than any pharmaceuticals including morphine." (KS).

TAPERING METH, CRACK, K2 AND COCAINE

Meth, crack, K2 and cocaine usually do not have strong physical withdrawals, but they do have mental withdrawals. Taper down and try using green strains to cope with the mental withdrawals and white for energy.

"Meth and crack don't have strong physical withdrawal symptoms; it is a psychological addiction. Fly high, crash and burn… Depression. I'm a recovering crack addict and I detoxed on my own. I used green mood enhancing and uplifting strains." (AF).

"Me and some family members used to be very, very addicted to K2 and it's horrible when you can't sleep or want it. I will tell you that Kratom is nothing like K2 but it'll help you get through cravings and withdrawals. That's what made me finally not need K2 anymore and stay off it." (HC).

"Kratom freed me from the meth monster." (SB).

"My son used greens and whites for meth cravings. Been clean a year now!" (CC).

"5 months off crack, Fentanyl and any mind-altering substance." (PB).

"Just started taking Kratom. It works good to wean off Meth, plus it's affordable and it doesn't control my life." (EB).

"I had major problems with K2 a little back. Kratom is all I need and I don't desire any drugs at all anymore. Kratom really helps with pain and staves off cravings. I even cut out marijuana with Kratom." (YC).

TAPERING ALCOHOL

If you have a high daily intake of alcohol don't just stop, taper down. Use beer to taper and gradually reduce intake over 3-7 days.

Avoid using Kratom if intoxicated with alcohol, it is not a good combination and you may get an adverse reaction or get physically sick. Kratom can help reduce cravings for alcohol for light and medium alcohol addictions. Maybe try using red sedative veins at night time and green anti-anxiety and antidepressant veins during daytime.

"I don't drink at all since I found Kratom and I used to drink pretty heavy! I have no desire at all for it!" (DS).

"From a man that used to live in the bottom of a bottle of Southern Comfort and drank at least a case of beer a day, I have had zero desire to drink alcohol since starting Kratom." (TV).

"I drank for the relief of anxiety, and Kratom pretty much takes care of that". (PS).

"I used to have a beer every night, now I skip nights, and if I do have one, I drink half, then pour the rest out. When I was on Methadone, I drank heavily and felt helpless to stop. With Kratom I have control". (JJ).

"I quit drinking alcohol with Kratom. Now I exercise and eat healthy food. No real withdrawals and no cravings. For 15 years I was drinking alcohol every day, equal to around ½ a bottle or more of hard liquor. I gradually stopped drinking alcohol (3-4 days), I started eating healthy food, take Kratom and do exercises every day. I had little anxiety and did not sleep through for a couple nights, but I was tired physically from the exercise, and that made me very relaxed. I have been offered alcohol almost daily since I quit but I have had no strong attraction to it, so, no alcohol at all. I am still in a state of shock, I was never able to quit alcohol in the past." (KB).

"Yes, 20 months sober from drinking". (DD).

"Yup I drank 15-30 beers every night for a solid 6 years". (SP).

"I have and it's the best thing I've ever done!!!" (CA).

"Yes absolutely! And I lost 15 pounds". (JB).

"I'm a recovering alcoholic. Since starting Kratom I have had no desire for a drink at all." (JF).

"I was a drunk for 20+ years and after being on Kratom for 6-8 months I just gradually lost the desire for alcohol! I didn't even try". (CK).

"From being a daily drinker (alcoholic) to maybe one or two on the weekend." (SP).

"6 months off subs! And today is 30 days off alcohol thanks to Kratom". (SE).

"I used to drink DAILY. Since taking Kratom I barely ever drink now. Just don't have the urge. I think I used to drink to self-medicate my anxiety. And Kratom helps me with that now". (BM).

If you are thinking about weaning off drugs or alcohol, you can eliminate the cravings, withdrawal symptoms and get a positive and optimistic perspective by using Kratom, while you rebuild your body with vitamins, minerals, detox, and exercise. You can get a new life.

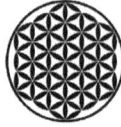

CHAPTER SIXTEEN

REDUCING THE INITIAL ADDICTION WITHDRAWAL SYMPTOMS

When reducing cravings and initial withdrawal symptoms for opioids, the method is, in general, the same no matter what addiction is left behind. Higher doses of Kratom in the beginning is how to reduce the cravings and withdrawal symptoms. After the first period of initial symptoms, Kratom should be tapered down, most likely it will happen automatically because the cravings and withdrawal symptoms decrease significantly.

"I used Kratom to wean off heroin, Oxycodone, Opana, Methadone, and Suboxone." (BG).

"I'm on day 7 with no Norco. I have cut my Kratom already and have had zero withdrawals from either. It's amazing stuff!" (TM).

Red veins are usually most effective to reduce withdrawal symptoms, cravings, pain and can be energetic or sedative.

For example, Red Maeng Da is an energetic daytime vein and Red Horn is a sedative evening/night vein. Green veins are usually most effective to reduce cravings, anxiety, panic attacks, pain, depressing thoughts and gives extra energy and uplifting mood.

"I used Red Bali and mixed it with whites and greens. I wasn't sick one day. I didn't miss one day of work. If you use it correctly it will work. It's scary to jump off that cliff and let the pills go. It is so worth it." (SO).

"6 grams of Red MD every 4 hours is all it took for me. For oxy it took about a week. For methadone it took about a month." (KA).

"The key is if you're feeling withdrawal symptoms—you need to take more Kratom! You will need more in the first 5–7 days (I took anywhere from 2 tsp—2 TBSP) every 2–6 hours (depending on how long it takes for your symptoms to begin to reappear) the first week. You'll be able to taper your dose tremendously after that." (MA).

"During the Suboxone wean off I took almost 2 tablespoons (mostly reds), every 4 hours for 2 weeks, then I tapered down the dose to 2 teaspoons, and so on, down to nothing". (GP).

"Reds are best for detox. I myself prefer Red Maeng Da for opiate withdrawal. One may need to dose a lot during the first couple weeks, I dosed about 2 teaspoons every 3–4 hours. It probably took away 75% + of my withdrawal symptoms." (TM).

"Love it. Best thing that ever happened to me. 3 grams red 3 to 4 times a day worked great. 3 months and 16 days clean. I was on 100 mg Fentanyl and 240 Oxycodone 30 a month for 13 years." (JG).

"On opiate detox…. Take more when you need it. Some people need as much as several tablespoons! But don't start out that high! For detox, a typical dose is 1-3 teaspoons every 2-4 hours. Take as much as you need now then slowly taper it back down in 4-6 weeks." (CC).

"Reds are best for pain and withdrawal. Get a few different reds so you can rotate. That way you won't get same strain syndrome. I add a green or white to my dose to help with mood and energy. I took 2 teaspoons every 3 hours. As soon as you feel the withdrawal coming back. Dose." (GM).

"Subutex wean off. I took 6-8 teaspoons a day. Usually 2 teaspoons every 3-4 hours for 4 weeks. Then I gradually went down over a year and stayed on 1 teaspoon or less a day for a few months and then stopped".

"When I stopped Subs I had to take 2 teaspoons every 2-3 hours for the first 3 weeks. Then I dropped to 1.5 for a month then up again. It comes in waves for some months."

"I used Red Vein during daytime and Red Bali when I quit Tramadol 2 months ago. I had to take a TBSP every 4-5 hours at first." (AA).

"I just came off Suboxone about 6 and a half months ago. During withdrawals take 1 to 2 teaspoons at a time and if

you don't feel anything in about an hour take, half teaspoon more as often as needed every few hours, I dosed more during withdrawals." (KO).

"I dose every 2-3 hours 2 tsp I put it in a little juice bottle I fill about 4 oz and mix my Kratom and chug it down." (VC).

"Red Kratom every 2-3 hours. Only withdrawal symptom was diarrhea. Got me off opiates fast." (LF).

"Take as much as you need. After a while you will automatically start dosing less frequently. I had to dose more often and higher doses while getting off Cymbalta. After 4 months I stopped having withdrawals and was able to cut back on Kratom drastically." (DK).

"I detoxed from 80-100 mgs opiates a day for 4 years, cold turkey. I had no choice but to hold on and ride it out. It can be done and it does suck. I personally used 1-3 teaspoons 3-5 times a day of red veined Kratom mixed with a 1/4 t of white and green veined to balance energy and mood." (AN).

"Days 1-3 I was dosing every 2/3 hours (1-2 tsp) days 4 and 5 I reduced by half and started dosing every 4 hours. But was able to sleep through the night. Wake up to dose every 2 hours." (LN).

"Day 7 and feeling better every day! If you are in doubt that Kratom helps for Suboxone withdrawals, I'll tell you now that IT CAN!!! I never imagined I could jump off this medicine and not be in misery for a couple of weeks but I'm a believer now!" (JH).

"Today was my day 12! After years of being on Norco's and Opana and then Suboxone, I did it!! I jumped from 6 mg and I'm never looking back thanks to this awesome plant. The past 10 days were not easy, I was exhausted and had insomnia and my brain felt like mush but I survived! On day 11 I started feeling pretty good and today made me feel like the withdrawals were a thing from the past! I'm truly a believer." (MM).

"Helped me kick a 140 Mg Methadone dose and I am finally free. No more rehabs, county jails or prisons. With Kratom, I am able to stay off Oxycodone and dope." (Anonymous).

"Kratom got me off almost 3 years of Methadone dependency. Kratom saved my life." (MC).

"6 months off Subs. I still experience withdrawals. (PAWS). I'm down to 1 tsp every 5 hours. At week 3 I was dosing every 2 hours 3-5 Tsp. Be patient, it takes time." (JD).

CHRONIC PAIN ILLNESS AND REDUCING OR WEANING OFF PRESCRIPTION MEDICATION WITH KRATOM

Some pain clinics earn their money selling pharmaceutical products. They may not be interested in a patient using Kratom because that patient may end up weaning of the pharmaceutical product and then they lose a patient. Some pain clinics test for Kratom and may terminate treatment. Patients equal money. Fortunately, some ethic pain clinics do suggest their patients use Kratom to reduce or wean off painkiller prescription medication.

Many people have used Kratom to dramatically reduce their use of prescription medication or have replaced it fully with Kratom using it in a responsible way. They have often done it gradually.

"I used reds last month to come off of pain pills. I just kept replacing the dose with powder until I was no longer taking the pills. I was serious about it. Now, this steroid withdrawal has been a bitch and schooled me in what withdrawing is like. Yesterday, I began to add a green (I have never done green or white) and it made all the difference. Took me from a flipping out anxiety, losing it, withdrawal to completely calm in 20 minutes. It was amazing. So, add a green." (KS).

"I take Kratom for chronic pain. I am not using any opiates, I have been free of them for 5 years. The opiate side effects were horrible for me. Kratom helps with my pain, more than anything else I am willing to take. It also rid me of insomnia, a relic of stopping opiate use. I do not get high, depressed, or crave drugs on Kratom". (R).

"It's possible, been taking Norco's for at least 11 years. Got some Kratom and haven't touched them since 8 days ago. I have 100 pills from my last refill just sitting there and I feel no craving or urge to take any". (LN).

"I've been on Opiates for pain for 10+ years. I have built up a tolerance and it is just taking the edge off the pain. I Just recently tried Kratom. I have not stopped prescription meds completely yet. I take pain meds first thing in the morning,

then later instead of a dose of prescription meds, I have taken Kratom. It seems to work so much better on my pain. I get stuff done now. I can't believe it and I'm afraid to believe it." (JD).

"I abruptly stopped 60 Mg Percocet and replaced it with Kratom. I have fibromyalgia, lupus, Sjogrens and back problems like herniated discs and endometriosis. I used Red Borneo and Red Thai when I did the switch. Both of these seem to work really well for my pain." (KD).

"Kratom helped me stop pain meds after 17 years of use for chronic pain conditions." (MC).

"I went from Norco 10's straight to Kratom and never had any withdrawals. Kratom rocks." (CN).

"I'm a 13 years opiate user and I went directly to Kratom. No withdrawals I feel great almost a month now." (KK).

"Thirty years of addiction. Fourteen months clean. It's indeed possible." (RH).

"One thing I've noticed since starting Kratom is I've had literally NO pain! Pain was my #1 reason for staying on morphine for 15 years!" (IJ).

"I went to a pain clinic for 10 years and I'm so glad I told them to kiss my little white ass. I'm on month 8 with just Kratom and feel SOOOOO much better. Most of all I don't have a 16th of the pain I had on opiates. (JH)."

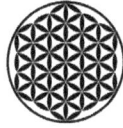

CHAPTER SEVENTEEN

DIET AND BRAIN HEALTH

"Recent evidence suggests that good nutrition is essential for our mental health and that a number of mental health conditions may be influenced by dietary factors." (https://www.mentalhealth.org.uk/a-to-z/d/diet-and-mental-health).

Weaning off various kinds of drugs, the mental withdrawal symptoms (here focus on anxiety and depression), happens because of a change in the brain and gut chemistry. The drug impact on endorphins, serotonin, and dopamine is huge. The endorphin and dopamine receptors in the brain don't get what they need, and the serotonin is also pushed out of balance. Nutrition is key and we will look into food that promotes and supports the natural development of dopamine, endorphin, and serotonin.

Replenish your body with vitamins and minerals.

Learn strategies on how to cope with anxiety, panic attacks, and depression; it is all linked together.

DOPAMINE, SEROTONIN, AND ENDORPHINS ARE NEUROTRANSMITTERS, THEY CARRY SIGNALS BETWEEN SYNAPSES IN THE BRAIN AND NERVE CELLS

When people, over time, have had a user/abuser relationship with prescription medication drugs related to pain, anxiety, panic attacks, depression, sleep problems and/or street drugs, the chemistry of the brain is changed. The brain is used to receiving high levels of the neurotransmitters dopamine, endorphins and serotonin, and have therefore created many more receptors in the brain. All three of them play a major role in natural wellbeing and happiness. If we have a healthy balance in dopamine, endorphins, and serotonin, it will strongly support us to overcome cravings, withdrawal symptoms, anxiety, panic attacks, and depression.

When a user decides to wean off, detox or reduce their drug use, they will experience the imbalance. Now the receptors are too many and they do not receive the level of neurotransmitters they are used to. This is the reason why people experience first cravings and then withdrawal symptoms. Now there is a lack of balance and the balance needs to be rebuilt naturally through foods rich in vitamins and minerals. It can take months to rebalance receptors in the brain again, but it is well worth it. Some people are genetically disposed to too high or too low levels of dopamine, endorphins or serotonin in their brain chemistry and need medication to balance it, while other people experience an imbalance created by the use of street drugs or prescription medication.

Dopamine: Is a neurotransmitter in the brain, but is also important in other areas of the body. Dopamine is related to motivation, mood, reward, pleasure, body movement, and focus, memory, and problem-solving. Lack of dopamine often leads to a feeling of low motivation, low self-esteem, boredom, lack of focus and the ability to cope with stress. Restless legs are a symptom of low dopamine.

"Dopaminergic pathways have been implicated in many disorders including but not limited to, OCD, depression and bipolar, ADHD, schizophrenia, eating disorders, Parkinson's, drug addiction, and other psychotic disorders in addition to schizophrenia. Although the role of dopamine is often debated and is not clear-cut, a lot of research does implicate dopamine in the pathophysiology of these disorders. (Peter Stroem, 2016 Quora.com)".

Serotonin: Is a neurotransmitter in the brain, but is also found in the digestive tract where it is created and synthesized by tryptophan. People with a bad diet living on processed foods and/or have a lack of vitamins and minerals tend to have a lack of balance in serotonin levels. Serotonin is related to sleep, muscle pain perception, appetite, wakefulness, attention, and sensory perception. It is believed by many researchers that a lack of serotonin can lead to depression, anxiety, panic attack and aggression, and that low serotonin levels might be related to the current epidemic of depression.

Endorphin: Is a neurotransmitter in the brain and is also distributed throughout the nervous system. Endorphins are related to pain reduction, reducing fear and stress. It also induces euphoria and motivation. Low levels of endorphins increase pain and are linked to fibromyalgia, for example, and other types of chronic pain. It is commonly known that the body produces endorphins in response to hard exercise.

After the initial wean-off period with withdrawal symptoms, the PAWS can be greatly reduced in the following months. A healthy diet including plenty of fresh-pressed juice with healthy vegetables and fruits can help balance the 3 neurotransmitters. It is simple to start rebuilding and rebalancing dopamine, endorphins and serotonin levels. A lot of it relates to exercise and healthy food, preferably organic fruits, organic vegetables, real natural cheese, and meat and butter from grass-fed animals. People who are deficient in natural vitamins and minerals get unbalanced and often sick mentally, emotionally and/or physically. Canned food, mac and cheese, and pizza won't do it. Precooked or prepared food has very little nutrients at all. Any added vitamins etc. are most likely synthetic. (Cheap vitamins and minerals added to food or bought at the supermarket are often synthetic). Synthetic vitamins and minerals cannot be processed properly and used by the body, so when people think they are getting vitamins and minerals they are actually being depleted.

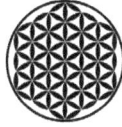

FOOD THAT PROMOTES AND SUPPORTS THE NATURAL DEVELOPMENT OF DOPAMINE, SEROTONIN AND ENDORPHINS

When using drugs, people get depleted from vitamins, minerals and nutrients. Often people don't care or are not aware of it. When addicted, three things happen. Avoiding withdrawal symptoms comes first and therefore medications/drugs comes before food, secondly the lack of appetite and third, drugs and alcohol often cause digestive problems. People don't get the vitamins and nutrition they need or spend time reflecting over healthy living. The answer is plenty of fresh vegetables, fruits, nuts, and exercise. You will notice that many different foods support all 3 neurotransmitters.

DOPAMINE

Foods that increase dopamine and are rich in vitamins and minerals:

- Raw or dark Chocolate
- Nuts
- Grass-fed beef, lamb, bison, and deer
- Dairy products and eggs from pasture-raised chicken
- Turkey
- Cauliflower
- Cabbage
- Brussel sprouts
- Chard
- Kale

SEROTONIN

You can increase your serotonin levels via the amino acid tryptophan which is a precursor for serotonin. It is known that tryptophan depletion is seen in people with mood disorders such as depression and anxiety.

Be aware that people low in serotonin often crave sugar and fat; you don't want that if your intention is to implement a healthy diet.

Foods which contain serotonin or increases serotonin and melatonin and are rich in vitamins and minerals:

- Nuts
- Bananas
- Pineapple
- Kiwis
- Tomato
- Plum
- Fermented foods
- High fat cold water fish
- Turmeric
- Green tea
- Raw or Dark Chocolate
- Tart cherries
- Oranges

Food rich in Tryptophan:

- Bananas
- Beets
- Grass-fed beef, lamb, bison, deer
- Dairy products and eggs from pasture raised chicken
- Turkey
- Oats
- Chickpeas
- Salmon and seafood in general
- Tofu

Other ways to increase melatonin:

Avoid all kind of light and WI-FI exposure in your bedroom at night, take a hot bath before going to bed, get outside and get sunlight every day.

"During her research at MIT Dr. Judith J. Wurtman discovered why people binge on sweets or starchy carbohydrates to relieve depression, anxiety, or anger. They do it because it raises their brain serotonin levels, thus making them feel happier." (bebrainfit.com). People on Methadone especially have problems with sweets, their teeth, and weight.

ENDORPHIN

There is no food which contains endorphins, but there are foods rich in vitamins and minerals which release, boost or stimulate the production of endorphins in the brain.

- Raw or Dark Chocolate
- Ginseng
- Oranges
- Chili peppers
- Spicy foods
- Strawberry
- Nuts
- All animal protein. Beef, poultry, and seafood

Natural ways to increase endorphins:

Exercise, dance, and yoga, massage, acupuncture, sex with your partner or solo, laughter and meditation can all individually increase the levels of endorphins in the body.

GABA

Gaba (gamma-aminobutanacid) is an important messaging neurotransmitter in the brain. Gaba reduces the activity of excited neurons and nerve cells. This directly impacts behavior, stress, and cognition. People diagnosed with depression, anxiety, panic attacks, insomnia, and PTSD often have low levels of Gaba. Gaba is not a direct food source, but some food can stimulate the production of Gaba naturally.

Food which stimulates natural Gaba production:

- Meat from grass-fed animals
- Eggs from pasture-raised animals
- Oily fish
- Raw organic dairy
- Tree nuts
- Seaweed
- Broccoli
- Spinach
- Tomatoes
- Mushrooms
- Whole grain oats, wheat etc.
- Lentils
- Brown rice
- Kefir
- Fermented foods

L-TYROSINE/TYROSINE

L-Tyrosine/Tyrosine is a strong amino acid that is a very important building block (synthesizer) for proteins, a precursor for the neurotransmitters dopamine, epinephrine, norepinephrine, and thyroid hormones. Moreover, tyrosine also helps the function of the adrenal and pituitary glands for production and regulating their hormones. Tyrosine supports mental health because it increases neurotransmitters, reduces stress and improves mood. People with depression due to a lack of balance in dopamine, epinephrine, and norepinephrine have experienced reduced depression and mood disorders when using tyrosine. Tyrosine is used to reduce withdrawal symptoms from heroin, cocaine, and alcohol.

Tyrosine is produced from the amino acid phenylalanine which is derived from food.

- Milk
- Eggs
- Cheese
- Fish
- Meat
- Nuts
- Beans
- Wheat
- Oats
- Bananas
- Avocado

FOODS THAT REDUCE INFLAMMATION

Inflammation leads to changes in the brain's ability to properly regulate hormones, and to changes in the production of neurotransmitters, such as serotonin and the ability to regenerate brain cells. Inflammation is linked to depression.

- Turmeric
- Ginger
- Garlic
- Nuts
- Oily fish
- Coffee
- Blueberries
- Oranges
- Cherries
- Tomatoes
- Leafy greens
- Extra virgin olive oil
- Apples
- Green tea
- Pau d'Arco tea
- Milk thistle
- Dandelion

All the various vitamins and minerals are essential for living a normal and healthy life. Just take a look at B12 for example. Vitamin B12 is a water-soluble vitamin with a key role in the normal functioning of the brain and nervous system, and for the formation of blood. A deficiency in vitamin B12 is related to OCD, mood disorders, psychosis, personality changes, loss of memory and depression. 30% of patients that are hospitalized for depression are deficient in vitamin B12. In general, all B vitamins are important for a well-functioning brain and a healthy nervous system.

Magnesium is a very important mineral for mental health. It reduces insomnia, anxiety, depression, fatigue, muscle cramps, high blood pressure, and irregular heartbeat. Magnesium is involved in more than 300 essential metabolic reactions in our body.

Zinc is another very essential mineral for brain health. A lack of zinc is linked to depressive behavior. Zinc has potential as a treatment for major depressive disorder.

Vitamin D deficiency is linked directly to depression.

Valium, Klonopin, Xanax, Clorazepate, and Ativan are known to deplete the body of melatonin which is important for sleep. In general, many antidepressants, mood stabilizers, Benzodiazepines, anticonvulsants, antipsychotic and central nervous stimulants deplete the body of many important vitamins and minerals. Symptoms of depletion of vitamins and minerals are similar to the many known side effects of various psychiatric medications.

Below are examples of some psychiatric medications that deplete the body of vitamins and minerals. Note that depletion of B12, magnesium, zinc and vitamin D result from most of the medications below.

ADDERALL depletes: Vitamin B12, vitamin C, and potassium.

PROZAK depletes: Vitamin B1, vitamin B2, vitamin B3, vitamin B6, vitamin B12, folic acid, vitamin C, vitamin D, coenzyme Q10, calcium, magnesium, manganese, selenium, sodium, zinc, and glutathione.

PAXIL depletes: Vitamin B1, vitamin B2, vitamin B3, vitamin B6, vitamin B12, folic acid, vitamin C, vitamin D, coenzyme Q10, calcium, magnesium, manganese, selenium, sodium, zinc, and glutathione.

ZOLOFT depletes: Vitamin B1, vitamin B2, vitamin B3, vitamin B6, vitamin B12, folic acid, vitamin C, vitamin D, coenzyme Q10, calcium, magnesium, manganese, selenium, sodium, zinc, and glutathione.

CELEXA depletes: Vitamin B1, vitamin B2, vitamin B3, vitamin B6, vitamin B12, folic acid, vitamin C, vitamin D, coenzyme Q10, calcium, magnesium, manganese, selenium, sodium, zinc, and glutathione.

WELLBUTRIN/ZYBAN depletes: Vitamin B6, vitamin C, vitamin D, coenzyme Q10, and sodium.

REMERON depletes: Vitamin B6, vitamin C, vitamin D, coenzyme Q10, and sodium.

EFFEXOR depletes: Vitamin B1, vitamin B2, vitamin B3, vitamin B6, vitamin B12, folic acid, vitamin C, vitamin D, coenzyme Q10, calcium, magnesium, manganese, selenium, sodium, zinc, and glutathione.

RISPERDAL depletes: Vitamin A, vitamin B1, vitamin B12, biotin, folic acid, carnitine, inositol, vitamin C, vitamin D, vitamin K, and calcium.

ZYPREXA depletes: Vitamin A, vitamin B1, vitamin B12, biotin, folic acid, carnitine, inositol, vitamin C, vitamin D, vitamin K, and calcium.

SEROQUEL depletes: Vitamin A, vitamin B1, vitamin B12, biotin, folic acid, carnitine, inositol, vitamin C, vitamin D, vitamin K, and calcium.

DEPAKOTE depletes: Vitamin A, vitamin B1, vitamin B2, vitamin B12, biotin, folic acid, carnitine, inositol, vitamin C, vitamin D, vitamin K, calcium, magnesium, and essential fatty acids.

(Antidepressants, antipsychotics and stimulants by Dr. David W. Tanton, Ph.D).

All vegetables and fruits have their place and so do seafood, organic grass-fed animals, poultry, and their products. Remember that the highest quality source of vitamins and minerals come from the source and real fruit and vegetables. Not from synthetic vitamins. Below is the FDA vitamin and mineral chart of the real food sources and vegetables and fruit.

Vitamins

VITAMIN	WHAT IT DOES	WHERE IS IT FOUND	DAILY VALUE*
Biotin	• Energy storage • Protein, carbohydrate, and fat metabolism	• Avocados • Cauliflower • Eggs • Fruits (e.g., raspberries) • Liver • Pork • Salmon • Whole grains	300 mcg
Folate/Folic Acid *Important for pregnant women and women capable of becoming pregnant*	• Prevention of birth defects • Protein metabolism • Red blood cell formation	• Asparagus • Avocado • Beans and peas • Enriched grain products (e.g., bread, cereal, pasta, rice) • Green leafy vegetables (e.g., spinach) • Orange juice	400 mcg
Niacin	• Cholesterol production • Conversion of food into energy • Digestion • Nervous system function	• Beans • Beef • Enriched grain products (e.g., bread, cereal, pasta, rice) • Nuts • Pork • Poultry • Seafood • Whole grains	20 mg
Pantothenic Acid	• Conversion of food into energy • Fat metabolism • Hormone production • Nervous system function • Red blood cell formation	• Avocados • Beans and peas • Broccoli • Eggs • Milk • Mushrooms • Poultry • Seafood • Sweet potatoes • Whole grains • Yogurt	10 mg
Riboflavin	• Conversion of food into energy • Growth and development • Red blood cell formation	• Eggs • Enriched grain products (e.g., bread, cereal, pasta, rice) • Meats • Milk • Mushrooms • Poultry • Seafood (e.g., oysters) • Spinach	1.7 mg
Thiamin	• Conversion of food into energy • Nervous system function	• Beans and peas • Enriched grain products (e.g., bread, cereal, pasta, rice) • Nuts • Pork • Sunflower seeds • Whole grains	1.5 mg

* The Daily Values are the amounts of nutrients recommended per day for Americans 4 years of age or older.

FDA http://www.fda.gov/nutritioneducation

Vitamins (cont'd)

VITAMIN	WHAT IT DOES	WHERE IS IT FOUND	DAILY VALUE*
Vitamin A	• Growth and development • Immune function • Reproduction • Red blood cell formation • Skin and bone formation • Vision	• Cantaloupe • Carrots • Dairy products • Eggs • Fortified cereals • Green leafy vegetables (e.g., spinach and broccoli) • Pumpkin • Red peppers • Sweet potatoes	5,000 IU
Vitamin B$_6$	• Immune function • Nervous system function • Protein, carbohydrate, and fat metabolism • Red blood cell formation	• Chickpeas • Fruits (other than citrus) • Potatoes • Salmon • Tuna	2 mg
Vitamin B$_{12}$	• Conversion of food into energy • Nervous system function • Red blood cell formation	• Dairy products • Eggs • Fortified cereals • Meats • Poultry • Seafood (e.g., clams, trout, salmon, haddock, tuna)	6 mcg
Vitamin C	• Antioxidant • Collagen and connective tissue formation • Immune function • Wound healing	• Broccoli • Brussels sprouts • Cantaloupe • Citrus fruits and juices (e.g., oranges and grapefruit) • Kiwifruit • Peppers • Strawberries • Tomatoes and tomato juice	60 mg
Vitamin D *Nutrient of concern for most Americans*	• Blood pressure regulation • Bone growth • Calcium balance • Hormone production • Immune function • Nervous system function	• Eggs • Fish (e.g., herring, mackerel, salmon, trout, and tuna) • Fish liver oil • Fortified cereals • Fortified dairy products • Fortified margarine • Fortified orange juice • Fortified soy beverages (soymilk)	400 IU
Vitamin E	• Antioxidant • Formation of blood vessels • Immune function	• Fortified cereals and juices • Green vegetables (e.g., spinach and broccoli) • Nuts and seeds • Peanuts and peanut butter • Vegetable oils	30 IU
Vitamin K	• Blood clotting • Strong bones	• Green vegetables (e.g., broccoli, kale, spinach, turnip greens, collards, Swiss chard, mustard greens)	80 mcg

* The Daily Values are the amounts of nutrients recommended per day for Americans 4 years of age or older.

FDA http://www.fda.gov/nutritioneducation

Minerals

MINERAL	WHAT IT DOES	WHERE IS IT FOUND	DAILY VALUE*
Calcium *Nutrient of concern for most Americans*	• Blood clotting • Bone and teeth formation • Constriction and relaxation of blood vessels • Hormone secretion • Muscle contraction • Nervous system function	• Almond, rice, coconut, and hemp milks • Canned seafood with bones (e.g., salmon and sardines) • Dairy products • Fortified cereals and juices • Fortified soy beverages (soymilk) • Green vegetables (e.g., spinach, kale, broccoli, turnip greens) • Tofu (made with calcium sulfate)	1,000 mg
Chloride	• Acid-base balance • Conversion of food into energy • Digestion • Fluid balance • Nervous system function	• Celery • Lettuce • Olives • Rye • Salt substitutes • Seaweeds (e.g., dulse and kelp) • Table salt and sea salt • Tomatoes	3,400 mg
Chromium	• Insulin function • Protein, carbohydrate, and fat metabolism	• Broccoli • Fruits (e.g., apple and banana) • Grape and orange juice • Meats • Spices (e.g., garlic and basil) • Turkey • Whole grains	120 mcg
Copper	• Antioxidant • Bone formation • Collagen and connective tissue formation • Energy production • Iron metabolism • Nervous system function	• Chocolate and cocoa • Crustaceans and shellfish • Lentils • Nuts and seeds • Organ meats (e.g., liver) • Whole grains	2 mg
Iodine	• Growth and development • Metabolism • Reproduction • Thyroid hormone production	• Breads and cereals • Dairy products • Iodized salt • Potatoes • Seafood • Seaweed • Turkey	150 mcg
Iron *Nutrient of concern for young children, pregnant women, and women capable of becoming pregnant*	• Energy production • Growth and development • Immune function • Red blood cell formation • Reproduction • Wound healing	• Beans and peas • Dark green vegetables • Meats • Poultry • Prunes and prune juice • Raisins • Seafood • Whole grain, enriched, and fortified cereals and breads	18 mg

* The Daily Values are the amounts of nutrients recommended per day for Americans 4 years of age or older.

FDA http://www.fda.gov/nutritioneducation

Minerals (cont'd)

MINERAL	WHAT IT DOES	WHERE IS IT FOUND	DAILY VALUE*
Magnesium	• Blood pressure regulation • Blood sugar regulation • Bone formation • Energy production • Hormone secretion • Immune function • Muscle contraction • Nervous system function • Normal heart rhythm • Protein formation	• Avocados • Bananas • Beans and peas • Dairy products • Green leafy vegetables (e.g., spinach) • Nuts and pumpkin seeds • Potatoes • Raisins • Wheat bran • Whole grains	400 mg
Manganese	• Carbohydrate, protein, and cholesterol metabolism • Cartilage and bone formation • Wound healing	• Beans • Nuts • Pineapple • Spinach • Sweet potato • Whole grains	2 mg
Molybdenum	• Enzyme production	• Beans and peas • Nuts • Whole grains	75 mcg
Phosphorus	• Acid-base balance • Bone formation • Energy production and storage • Hormone activation	• Beans and peas • Dairy products • Meats • Nuts and seeds • Poultry • Seafood • Whole grain, enriched, and fortified cereals and breads	1,000 mg
Potassium *Nutrient of concern for most Americans*	• Blood pressure regulation • Carbohydrate metabolism • Fluid balance • Growth and development • Heart function • Muscle contraction • Nervous system function • Protein formation	• Bananas • Beet greens • Juices (e.g., carrot, pomegranate, prune, orange, and tomato) • Milk • Oranges and orange juice • Potatoes and sweet potatoes • Prunes and prune juice • Spinach • Tomatoes and tomato products • White beans • Yogurt	3,500 mg
Selenium	• Antioxidant • Immune function • Reproduction • Thyroid function	• Eggs • Enriched pasta and rice • Meats • Nuts (e.g., Brazil nuts) and seeds • Poultry • Seafood • Whole grains	70 mcg

* The Daily Values are the amounts of nutrients recommended per day for Americans 4 years of age or older.

FDA http://www.fda.gov/nutritioneducation

Minerals (cont'd)

MINERAL	WHAT IT DOES	WHERE IS IT FOUND	DAILY VALUE*
Sodium *Nutrient to get less of*	• Acid-base balance • Blood pressure regulation • Fluid balance • Muscle contraction • Nervous system function	• Breads and rolls • Cheese (natural and processed) • Cold cuts and cured meats (e.g., deli or packaged ham or turkey) • Mixed meat dishes (e.g., beef stew, chili, and meat loaf) • Mixed pasta dishes (e.g., lasagna, pasta salad, and spaghetti with meat sauce) • Pizza • Poultry (fresh and processed) • Sandwiches (e.g., hamburgers, hot dogs, and submarine sandwiches) • Savory snacks (e.g., chips, crackers, popcorn, and pretzels) • Soups • Table salt	2,400 mg
Zinc	• Growth and development • Immune function • Nervous system function • Protein formation • Reproduction • Taste and smell • Wound healing	• Beans and peas • Beef • Dairy products • Fortified cereals • Nuts • Poultry • Seafood (e.g., clams, crabs, lobsters, oysters) • Whole grains	15 mg

* The Daily Values are the amounts of nutrients recommended per day for Americans 4 years of age or older.

FDA http://www.fda.gov/nutritioneducation

CHAPTER NINETEEN

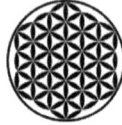

BODY DETOXIFICATION AND BODY REBUILDING

You are one decision from a life-changing lifestyle change. Eat healthy, exercise and stay hydrated must be your new motto. Maybe for too long, your diet has been less nutritious than it should be. Lack of vitamins and minerals have a direct impact on your wellbeing and your brain chemistry. It is also very important for the healing process of your body. The fastest way to replenish your body with vitamins, minerals, enzymes, and detox is juicing. Juice will flush toxins from tissues and muscles to the liver. The liver then needs help to detox the toxins out of the body. Coffee enemas are exceptionally good at detoxing the liver. More on coffee enemas later.

I start my day with 32 ounces of juice. If a juice has a lot of greens, it can be a little sour and hard for the digestive system so I add 2 apples. An apple a day keeps the doctor away; two apples may keep the doctor at a long distance. The best you can do is to use organic vegetables and fruits; they have no pesticide residue.

Juice ingredients can include:

- 2 tablespoons of apple cider vinegar
- ¼ teaspoon Himalayan pink salt
- 2 apples
- 3 carrots
- A chunk of ginger
- 1 tomato
- A handful of green beans (blanched)
- A quarter red, yellow or green sweet pepper
- A half head of romaine lettuce
- A handful of spinach
- 3-4 broccoli stalks, asparagus or kale
- Some red or white cabbage
- A handful of bean sprouts
- A quarter beet or some beet tops

PURIUM

If juice is not an option for you and you decide to take vitamins and minerals instead, then make sure it is organic whole food vitamins and minerals, these are made of real vegetables and fruit. They are not synthetic.

Juicing fresh vegetables and fruits can be both costly and time-consuming.

When I don't have funds to buy fresh produce or time to juice, I use Purium. Purium is an amazing product and is the perfect alternative as it comes as close as possible to real fresh pressed vegetables and fruits. The enzymes are still alive and active and the vitamins and minerals are not destroyed or harmed. This is superfood at the highest level.

The plants used in Purium grow in clean, mineral-rich soil and watered with clean mineral-rich water—no chemicals, herbicides or pesticides. No artificial colors, flavors, sweeteners, binders, fillers, hormones, non-irradiated and absolutely no genetically-modified ingredients. Nearly 100% of the fresh plant is converted into stable powder that can last for up to 2 years.

If you go to: ishoppurium.com and use the code Flower of Life you get $50 off your first order, minimum order is $75. If you return the next month you get 25% off, if you return only once every couple month you get 15% off. No auto shipping.

Purium also has high quality CDB oil 1500mg and the Flower of Life code can be used there as well. Go to: puriumcbd.com

When you stay focused and present with what you are doing in the NOW, like preparing a healthy meal, then you are not in the past and you are not in the future, you basically redirect your energy and thoughts to something which is good for you and your family.

Make sure that you drink plenty of water or coconut water which contains electrolytes. Stay hydrated, liquid helps flush out toxins from your tissues.

Many drug and alcohol users often have a damaged liver or damaged kidneys. This is often from the use of over-the-counter painkillers, prescription medication, illegal street drugs, or various diseases spread in various ways. How can you win a battle if you are not fit to fight? You will want to do the best to heal your internal organs; you need them for the rest of your life.

> "I know some of you with or without fatty liver are worried that Kratom may mess with your liver, but I just got my liver enzyme/function test results today and they all came back NORMAL. Since I started using Kratom, I have NEVER had another abnormal liver test result as I did years ago when I abused oxys and vics combined with acetaminophen. That being said, this is proof that Kratom is safer than Tylenol. I have fatty liver (due to past drug abuse, poor diet, being middle-aged and overweight), yet my liver enzymes have stayed within the NORMAL range during these past 2 years I have been using Kratom. Kratom also successfully got me away from a 3 years Suboxone addiction, too. It's truly a great feeling." (AM).

> "I have used Kratom daily for more than a year, eaten healthy and exercised. I just had my blood test done. All and everything improved, including liver enzymes. I don't think Kratom affected my liver in a bad way." (DM).

Milk thistle and dandelion are two amazing natural supplements which will help to detox, regenerate and heal your liver. Coffee enemas will help the body to eliminate toxins.

MILK THISTLE

Milk Thistle is an amazing plant when it comes to protecting and rebuilding the liver from damage. It is amazing for detoxing because it absorbs many different chemicals (pharmaceutical drugs, etc.), that otherwise would be dangerous and poisoning the body. Milk thistle can help to stop and reverse chronic fatty liver disease (cirrhosis). It helps to rebuild the liver.

Milk Thistle is also a strong antioxidant which fights inflammation and stimulates cells to regenerate and repair themselves, including the liver, joints and muscles. It furthermore stimulates the immune system, reduces cholesterol and helps balance insulin.

DANDELION

Dandelion is another amazing plant which can help to detox and regenerate the liver. Like Milk Thistle, dandelion supports bile flow. Bile contains the toxins which are being released from the liver. Dandelion can reduce blood pressure and helps regulate cholesterol as well. It also stimulates insulin production and supports regulation of blood sugar. Dandelions are rich in Vitamin A, Vitamin C, iron and calcium. Dandelion is diuretic so it helps release toxic build up in the kidneys.

COFFEE ENEMAS

Max Gerson (October 18, 1881—March 8, 1959) was a very wise man. He made the Gerson Protocol and people following his detox/healing protocol (based on juicing, organic fruits, vegetables, supplements and coffee enemas) often go from terminal illness to being healed. He said that toxins build up in body tissue, and eating a healthy vegetarian diet and doing body detox, will flush the toxins to the liver. To avoid toxic build up in the liver, the liver needs some help to get rid of the toxins. Coffee enema is one answer to that question. When the coffee is held in the colon for 12+ minutes it will help the liver to squeeze waste and toxins out. The coffee will also help flush out years' old waste from the colon. So, it is a win-win situation and it is very healthy. You might find it a bit weird the first few times if you are not used to it, but for sure it is well worth it; it will exercise and detox your liver.

Coffee enemas have been used to increase health for more than 500 years. It has been used to treat various illnesses from depression to cancer.

How Do Coffee Enemas Work?

Toxins are everywhere. They're in the food we eat, the water we drink, and the air we breathe and the medication we might take. So, it's crucial that we help our bodies to detox. Coffee enemas are one of the most effective methods of detoxing.

Coffee enemas stimulate the bile ducts, causing them to open and release toxic bile into the intestinal tract where it can leave the body instead of being reused and the toxins reabsorbed.

Juice flushes the tissue for toxins and takes it to the liver. The liver then needs help to release the toxins. Not only will coffee enemas help the liver to let go of toxins, it also cleanses the colon of waste. Since we are born, toxins have layered in our colon year after year. The toxins are still in there, releasing and they might have a big impact on our physical, mental and emotional health. Toxic build up in the body may cause pain and can be relieved with coffee enemas.

Coffee enemas also help clean the colon of bacteria, parasites, worms and candida yeast. All four of them can wreak serious havoc in our bodies when not balanced, treated or removed. If we don't have a healthy diet supporting healthy bacteria in our body, then harmful bacteria in our intestines will take over and they can induce or create anxiety, confusion, and depression.

When the body is free of toxins it can fully focus on healing and fight any disease that might come around.

Coffee is a high-level antioxidant which fights inflammation. Remember that inflammation leads to changes in the brain's ability to properly regulate hormones and changes in the production of neurotransmitters such as serotonin and the ability to regenerate brain cells. Inflammation is linked to depression.

Coffee contain vitamins and minerals. B2, B3, B5, calcium, manganese, potassium, zinc and magnesium are absorbed through the colon wall.

What do you need for a coffee enema?

Coffee, enema bucket, doggie pad or towel, lubricant.

How to do a Coffee enema:

Always use organic coffee if possible. Conventionally grown coffee has pesticide residue. Gerson recommend a quart-size for a coffee enema. Use a pot to boil the coffee, measure how much coffee/water you need (1, 2, or 3 quarts), add a proper amount of coffee to the water. Bring it to a boil and simmer it for 15 minutes. Let it cool to body temperature when doing a coffee enema. Lie on the right side and hold in the coffee for as long as you can, not less than 4 minutes and preferably 12 minutes. If pain due to air is experienced it often helps to lie on the back or to move the belly so the air can move. After 12 minutes or so, go to the toilet and release.

Some coffee is absorbed in the colon so do a coffee enema early during the day, then the coffee will not affect your sleep.

EXERCISE

"I am whole, perfect, strong, powerful, loving, harmonious and happy. (Haanel).

One of the best things you can do for yourself anytime is exercise. It will help heal and regenerate your body, mind and emotional being. It will also help prevent possible illness in the future, especially if Kratom and DLPA have eliminated the withdrawal symptoms and exercise is now combined with a healthy diet. The time is NOW and you can do it. Your body has an amazing ability to relatively quickly heal and regenerate. Some scientists say that we, on the cellular level, regenerate the body within a year. Even if you have lived years with an improper diet you can still reverse and regenerate much damage within 6-12 months. That is a very low price to pay for increasing your well-being physically, mentally and emotionally, and also adding on many more years to your life span. When you get started with exercise, detox and a healthy diet it will take you to a place you thought impossible and only dreamt about. It is possible. Persist and you will be rewarded greatly.

"Conclusive evidence exists that physical inactivity is an important cause of most chronic diseases. In addition, physical activity primarily prevents, or delays, chronic diseases, implying that chronic disease need not be an inevitable outcome during life". (Frank Booth, Ph.D., Christian Roberts, Ph.D., Matthew Laye, Ph.D. nih.gov, 2014.).

"The more exercise people do, the lower their social anxiety". (Dr. Matthew Willmire).

"I'm also a huge advocate for working out...it's so good, not only for physical health, but mental health as well, and with regular exercise, it decreases cravings and anxiety,

and in the short-term, it boosts your mood and energy levels tremendously! Also it's a good thing to do while you wait for a craving to pass, or to combat an anxiety/panic attack...I've been told for years by so many people to exercise to help my anxiety and depression but could never get motivated...I've been working out for 90 min a day and 6 days a week since August and I consider it to be a major factor in how well I am managing my mental health and staying on track with sobriety, not to mention losing all the weight is a plus."
(HA).

"Rumor has it you can replace one addiction for another. I'd rather look beastly than strung out though. Exercise." (GG).

"Now I'm really seeing results and leaving my addiction behind. Exercise is truly amazing." (LS).

"Totally agree. Thanks to the gym I was also able to quit taking antidepressants." (AM).

This book is being read by many people, some with chronic diseases or disabilities. I will not put up any exercise schemes in this book. I will suggest that you, yourself, who knows if you have any physical limitations, start exercising daily and then add on within your physical ability. Don't overdo it but increase over time whatever exercises you decide to do. Mix walking with running, bike for miles or swim 10, 20, 30, 40 laps or more. Use machines in your own home, go to the gym, go to the beach, go to the forest. Do it daily or as often you can. Don't be cozy or too comfortable. Go out of your comfort zone. Push your boundaries; this is about you weaning off opioids, street drugs or prescription medications. Your life is the treasure and your reward. This is about surviving and creating a pleasant life for yourself and your family.

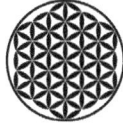

CHAPTER TWENTY

ADDITIONAL OVER-THE-COUNTER PRODUCTS

For people who don't like Kratom or can't achieve the benefits of Kratom, there are other products which can reduce withdrawals. These over-the-counter products can also be used together with Kratom to ease any withdrawal symptoms.

Amino acids are used in addiction recovery to help create new neurotransmitters and help the brain to rebuild and rebalance.

Ishoppurium.com has an cminent Amino acid blend 5000 mg:

L-Leucine, L-Lysine HCL, L-Valine, L-Isoleucine, L-Phenylalanine DLPA, L-Threonine, L-Methionine, L-Tryptophan.

Go to Ishoppurium.com and use the Flower of Life code and get $50 off of your first order of a minimum order of $75.

DLPA

DLPA is a combination of two forms of amino acids. D-phenylalanine and L-phenylalanine. Both of them are important for a variety of functions in our brain and nervous system, and in our body in general. D-phenylalanine is found in some protein-rich food but only in small amounts. D-phenylalanine is synthesized in laboratories.

> *"I highly recommend DLPA for anyone who wants to taper off and/or quit cold turkey. The stuff works wonders. For me, it completely took my craving away. It boosts my mood. As far as withdrawal-wise, the only thing I'm going thru is small leg aches. Nothing too bad at all." (DT).*

> *"DLPA has really been helping with my mood from withdrawals." (DP).*

The L-phenylalanine is found in protein-rich food and is known to help the brain to produce neurotransmitters like epinephrine, norepinephrine, and dopamine. In an open study dl-phenylalanine, in doses from 75-200 mg/day, was administered to 20 depressed patients for 20 days. At the end of the trial, 12 patients (8 with complete, 4 with good response) were discharged without any further treatment. 4 patients with partially untypical depressions experienced mild to moderate responses, whereas 4 patients did not respond at all to the phenylalanine administration. (https://www.ncbi.nlm.nih.gov/pubmed/335027).

In a double-blind study, alcoholics who were treated with DLPA, nutrients, and multivitamins had reduced withdrawal symptoms and reduced stress. (http://www.uofmhealth.org/health-library/hn-2895002).

Recommended dosage is considered to be from 50-500mg daily. However, some websites do suggest that users may benefit from taking up to 1000mg a day for a temporary period of time.

DLPA is known to reduce depression, increase energy, improve cognitive function and reduce pain.

DLPA can increase high blood pressure and interact with medication. If you take medication you should consult your medical supplier. If you have high blood pressure maybe start at a low dose, like 100mg a day. Increase the dose slowly and under a medical suppliers supervision.

5-HTP (5-HYDROXYTRYPTOPHAN)

5-HTP is an important amino acid and is related to serotonin production. 5-HTP can help reduce anxiety, depression and insomnia. Anxiety and depression are often linked to low levels of serotonin. 150—400 mg daily can help increase serotonin. Read the information on food which increase serotonin and tryptophan. Long-Term supplementation with 5-HTP can deplete dopamine, norepinephrine, and epinephrine, so use 5-HTP supplements temporarily during withdrawals with caution. Some medications used during surgery can increase serotonin levels. Stop using 5-HTP supplements 2 weeks before a scheduled surgery.

GABA (GAMMA-AMINOBUTYRIC ACID)

Gaba supplements are most often synthetic. Gaba reduce depression, anxiety, panic attacks, insomnia and PTSD. People diagnosed with depression, anxiety, panic attacks insomnia and PTSD often have very low levels of Gaba. 250—650 mg 3 times a day.

MAGNESIUM

As mentioned earlier, magnesium is a very important mineral for mental health. It reduces insomnia, anxiety, depression, fatigue, muscle cramps, high blood pressure and irregular heartbeat. Magnesium is involved in more than 300 essential metabolic reactions in our body.

"Magnesium was found usually effective for treatment of depression in general use. Related and accompanying mental illnesses in these case histories including traumatic brain injury, headache, suicidal ideation, anxiety, irritability, insomnia, postpartum depression, cocaine, alcohol and tobacco abuse, hypersensitivity to calcium, short-term memory loss, and IQ loss were also benefited. The possibility that magnesium deficiency is the cause of most major depression and related mental health problems including IQ loss and addiction is enormously important to public health." (https://www.ncbi.nlm.nih.gov/pubmed/16542786/).

During a drug wean-off there are several things besides Kratom which can help alleviate RLS (Restless Legs Syndrome) withdrawal symptoms. Caleb Treeze Organic Farm RLS (the old Amish remedy), Hyland's Restful Legs, multivitamins, especially whole food supplements or iron-rich vegetables. Many drug users have very low iron levels. Drink plenty of water. Magnesium, warm showers and Epsom salt baths. Massage, stretching, exercise and a pillow between your legs during nighttime can help as well. Very important is the potassium levels. Potassium deficiency will make you feel wiped out, experience spasms and weak crampy muscles, increased heartbeat, dizziness, tingling and annoying pins and needles sensations.

You can see in the FDA vitamin and mineral chart which foods contain potassium, magnesium and iron.

Most of the following natural supplements are very often used by people weaning off opioids, street drugs, and prescription medications because these supplements help reduce anxiety, depression, pain, insomnia, stress, cramps and inflammation, and therefore also reduce various withdrawal symptoms. All these supplements have many more qualities related to natural healing and general health than just those mentioned. Many synthetic pharmaceutical medications mimic the qualities of these natural herbs and plants. Here we mostly focus on the qualities which reduce withdrawal symptoms, PAWS, benefit addiction recovery in general and can help rebuild physical, emotional, mental and spiritual well-being. Read all about them and take them into consideration. Herbs and supplements in general are regulated as food, not drugs, by the United States Food and Drug Administration (FDA). They can be used in combination with Kratom or without

Kratom to reduce initial withdrawal symptoms and PAWS while you rebuild dopamine, serotonin, endorphins, vitamins, and minerals with natural healthy food. **You got this!**

MAGNOLIA BARK (MAGNOLIA OFFICINALIS)

Magnolia is a plant native to Asia and is an important part of Chinese and Tibetan herbal medicine. Magnolia is known to help reduce anxiety, depression, insomnia, inflammation and pain caused by inflammation. Magnolia increase serotonin and noradrenaline. Anxiety, depression and mania are often linked to low levels of serotonin. 200—800 mg daily or 2/3 teaspoon of powder. Don't use Magnolia during pregnancy, stop using Magnolia 2 weeks prior to scheduled surgery and consult your doctor if you have a bleeding disorder.

INCARVILLEA SINESIS

Incarvillea is a plant native to Asia and is an important part of traditional Chinese and Mongolian herbal medicine. Incarvillea is known to reduce anxiety, insomnia, restlessness, pain, rheumatism, cramps and inflammation. Use as advised or if using powder, 5—15 g cooked in water.

CORDYCEPS SINESIS

Cordyceps is a mushroom native to altitudes over 14.000 feet. Cordyceps is an important part of ancient Chinese and

Tibetan herbal medicine. Cordyceps is known to improve sleeping patterns, energy and endurance and is used by many athletes. Cordyceps also help detox the body, is anti-aging, strengthens the immune system and balances cholesterol levels. 1000—3000 mg or ¼ to ½ teaspoon powder daily is recommended. It can be used in smoothies, water, tea or coffee. Cordyceps lowers glucose levels, if you are diabetic, have an immune disorder or a bleeding disorder you should consult your doctor or avoid using cordyceps.

KAVA (PIPER METHYSTICUM)

Kava is a plant native to the western Pacific Islands. It is known to reduce anxiety, depression, insomnia, stress, restlessness and muscle pain. It is also used to reduce withdrawals from benzodiazepines. Kava works on Dopamine and GABA receptors in the brain. 1 teaspoon or 2 powder in a glass of water. If you have a liver disease consult with your doctor before using Kava. Kava used in combination with Xanax or sedatives may cause excessive drowsiness.

AKUAMMA SEEDS

Akuamma seeds comes from the Picralima Nitida tree. It is native to tropical climates and is an important part especially of African herbal medicine. Akuamma is especially known for its strong pain reducing qualities, reducing anxiety and stress, and can reduce opioid withdrawals. It is often used by people suffering from anxiety and stress, chronic pain and symptoms related to fibromyalgia, herniated discs, back pain in general and sports injuries. Akuamma reduce inflammation. A daily dosage is 1/3 teaspoon of freshly grounded powder for maximum benefits. 2-5 grams is the range of general use, or suck on a seed or 2 for 30 minutes till it gets soft. Powder can be used to make tea, combined with food or in capsules.

LEMON BALM (MELISSA OFFICINALIS)

Lemon balm is a herb used in ancient traditional folk medicine around the world. Lemon balm helps reduce anxiety, panic attacks, depression, insomnia, pain, rapid heartbeat and inflammation. Lemon balm help increase cognitive performance and the positive qualities of GABA in the brain. It helps reduce stress and induce calmness and is mood enhancing. It helps lower blood sugar. Lemon balm should not be taken in combination with sedative prescription medication. Use as advised or if using powder, 1/3 of a teaspoon daily.

PASSION FRUIT (PASSIFLORA INCARNATE)

Passion fruit is used to make medicine. It is a sedative and is known to reduce anxiety, insomnia, depression, pain, muscle spasms, irregular heartbeat, high blood pressure and symptoms related to narcotic withdrawal. Use as advised or if using powder, 1 -2 grams equal to ¼ teaspoon.

MARIJUANA (CANNABIS)

The use of marijuana for religious, medicinal and recreational purposes goes 5000 years back. Many people who wean off opioids and pharmaceutical medical prescription addictions in general use marijuana for its medicinal qualities.

However, there are a couple things to pay attention to. Cannabis basically has 2 different main strains. Sativa which mostly affects the mind (psychoactive) and Indica which mostly affects the body. Hybrids are a combination of both strains and their qualities. All 3 of them contain THC and CBD. The level of THC and CBD plays a role in how strong the effect is. People prone to anxiety may not want to use pure Sativa and especially not with a high THC levels, it can give an unpleasant psychoactive experience, while Indica may give them bodily relaxation. For people who don't want the psychoactive experience, Indica or CBD products is preferred.

Cannabis Sativa has higher levels of THC. Sativa is typically uplifting, energetic, induce creativity and social behavior. Sativa reduces chronic pain, migraines and nausea.

Cannabis Indica has higher levels of CBD. Indica is typically relaxing and calming. Indica reduces insomnia, anxiety, chronic pain, muscle spasms and stress.

Cannabis THC products are legal for medicinal purposes or recreational use in some states. Cannabis can be tolerance-building or addictive when not used with awareness. If inexperienced with cannabis, start at low THC levels and low dose.

CBD OR CANNABIDIOL (CANNABIS)

CBD or cannabidiol is derived from Marijuana/Cannabis. Cannabinoid receptors are a part of the human body and are located throughout the body in the brain, nervous system, liver, lungs and kidneys. CBD is helping the brain and nervous system repair after injury or damage.

CBD can be used as tincture, oil, cream, edibles or It can be vaped. Scientific research indicate that CBD can reduce anxiety, depression, sleep problems, epilepsy (anti-seizure), chronic pain, inflammation, heart disease and other benefits. Pure CBD oil is NOT psychoactive and is well known and very popular among people in rehabilitation.

RHODIOLA ROSEA

Rhodiola is a plant native to colder mountainous regions in Scandinavia, Russia, Europe and Asia. Rhodiola is used to treat anxiety, depression, stress, fatigue and exhaustion. It is slightly stimulating. 300—600 mg or less (1/10th of a teaspoon powder).

ASHWAGANDA (WITHANIA SOMINIFERA)

Ashwaganda is plant widely used in ancient ayurvedic medicine as an all-around herbal medicine. Aswaganda reduces anxiety, stress, cortisol and pain. Ashwaganda is anti-inflammatory, antibacterial, antiparasitic, antiviral and antifungal. It protects the heart, liver and kidneys and enhances brain function and memory.

It is used to reduce withdrawal symptoms. Use as advised or if using powder, ½ to 1 teaspoon powder daily is recommended.

ST. JOHN'S WORT (HYPERICUM PERFORATUM)

St. John's wort is an ancient medical plant used for more than 2000 years. St. John's wort is known to reduce anxiety, depression, mood swings, stress, pain, OCD, sleep problems and reduce withdrawal symptoms. St. John's wort is anti-inflammatory, antiviral and is rich in antioxidants. It is a natural remedy often recommended by psychiatrists and doctors because it is believed to help the brain produce more dopamine, serotonin and norepinephrine. It is considered equivalent to Clonidine. St. John's wort does interact with some medications (SSRIs, anticonvulsants, Xanax) and can possibly reduce their effectiveness. If you use any of the above mentioned or are diagnosed with bipolar disorder or schizophrenia you should consult your doctor before using St. John's wort. 300 mg 2-3 times a day.

VALERIAN (VALERIANA OFFICINALIS)

Valerian is a very popular ancient natural remedy for reducing insomnia, anxiety, emotional stress and muscle tensions. Valerian is often used as a supplement by people weaning off Benzodiazepines and antidepressants. Powder, tea or capsules. 400-900 mg 1 hour before bedtime.

MORINGA (MORINGA OLEIFERA)

Moringa is a very popular natural remedy used in ancient Ayurvedic, Greek, Egypt and Roman herbal medicine. Moringa is power packed with phytonutrients, protein, vitamins, minerals and essential amino acids. It contain vitamin A, vitamin B1, B2, B3, B6, folate, vitamin C, calcium, potassium, iron, magnesium, phosphorus and zinc. Moringa is antifungal, anti-inflammatory, antiviral and antidepressant. Moringa protects the liver and kidneys. It balances blood pressure and cholesterol levels. It treats stomach disorders and can reduce constipation. Moringa is beneficial for hair, skin and bones. It is used to treat arthritis and it is also used to treat neurodegenerative diseases because it can help restore brain monoamines, (dopamine, serotonin and norepinephrine). Don't use Moringa during pregnancy. The powder can be used in cooking and smoothies etc. There is no maximum dosage but it is recommended to start with ½—1 teaspoon.

MELATONIN

Is a hormone produced naturally in our body that regulates our sleep-wake cycle. When we get older melatonin production often decrease. Melatonin is synthetic made but some natural food sources contain melatonin or can help produce melatonin. See the information on natural food which contain serotonin or increases serotonin and melatonin. Natural or synthetic melatonin reduce insomnia, sleep problems, restless legs and increase REM sleep, immune function and regulates appetite and digestion. For sleep problems 2—3 mg 30 minutes before bedtime is recommended.

Synthetic melatonin may interact with prescription sedatives, antidepressants, anticonvulsants and antipsychotics. It may be a good idea to avoid these combinations and it is best to avoid using melatonin during pregnancy, breastfeeding, depression and if you have a bleeding disorder. Consult your doctor first if you are in doubt or eat natural food instead of synthetic melanin.

HYDROXIZINE (VISTARIL, ATARAX)

Hydroxizine is used to reduce nausea, itching and anxiety. It's basically Benadryl which is non-addictive. Don't feel bad about taking it temporarily, especially if you need it. It is given to people in rehab. Follow the guidelines.

IMODIUM (LOPERAMIDE)

Imodium reduces diarrhea, cramps, pressure, bloating and gas. Make sure you follow the guidelines.

HYLAND'S RESTFUL LEGS

Hyland's restful legs reduces restlessness, jerking, twitching, urgent to move and tingling. Follow the guidelines.

Tonic water contain quinine which reduce muscle cramps. 8 oz before bedtime.

Lots of really warm baths. Epsom salt can be used in the bathtub.

Freshly made ginger tea, ginger and gingerade are great to reduce nausea.

If you choose to go through withdrawals without Kratom you may want to fill your day with something to redirect attention from withdrawal symptoms to something else.

Regardless of whether you have a DVD player, Netflix or Youtube, make sure you watch positive movies and inspirational videos on detoxing your body, nutrition, guided meditations, how to juice and how to exercise, however you like to exercise. Change bad habits to new good habits.

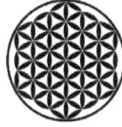

CHAPTER TWENTY-ONE

HOW I COPED WITH ANXIETY, PANIC ATTACKS AND DEPRESSION WITHOUT USING PHARMACEUTICAL DRUGS

Anxiety and panic attacks are very unpleasant to deal with. Anxiety starts, then a panic attack might take over, and we think we are dying because we lose control over our body and thoughts. We don't die, and we can cope with anxiety and a panic attack without taking pharmaceuticals. Drugs numb our emotions and feelings; without drugs, we now experience reality (and everything in it) again. For a period of time, it makes us hyper-aware and super sensitive. It is a process and it is temporary. It takes time to go through the process, step by step and it is possible.

In my past, I myself went through a period of anxiety, panic attacks and depression. At that time, I did not have Kratom's anti-anxiety and anti-depression qualities to help me, but I will share about it because it might inspire somebody. I went through various fears and phobias like pearls on a string. Fear of losing control, panic attacks, being alone, with other people, shopping for food, standing in line, in the mall, in the elevator, in the bus, in the train, on the airplane, of being sick, of no way out and of dying. No matter how intense my experience or my negative thoughts were, suicide was never an option.

I managed to work my way through anxiety, panic attack and depression without ever using any kind of pharmaceuticals at all. It was sometimes very intense and my way through was by changing diet, exercise and developing techniques. The following techniques described later are for inspiration. It took me about a year. In the beginning, the anxiety and panic attacks increased; I kept in mind that people don't die from a panic attack. One day it topped off, I surrendered, and from that day on they decreased. Less anxiety and each panic attack then became shorter and less intense and the time in between them became longer and longer. One day they stopped. If any thought, kind of anxiety or bodily sensation happened, which in the past would have ignited a full-blown panic attack, I now had my techniques. And it would not happen. Over time you can learn how to cope with it and then you become in control. Take your power back, it belongs to you. You can create a new life for yourself. **You got this!**

MY STORY

20 years ago, way before I heard about Kratom, I went through hell myself. (My father died; my grandparents died. I had a serious accident and ended up with severe pain. I lost

my well-paid job. I lost my relationship. I lost my apartment to foreclosure,...and my mother went into a deep black hole with addictions after my father died. I love my mom and for many years I tried to help her and be there for her, but it was an uphill battle.

After my father died, my mother began to use alcohol. During her treatment, she was prescribed and used Benzodiazepines and SSRIs. These are the side effects I witnessed:

I quickly noticed that even after my mother was using Benzodiazepines and SSRI medication, she was still anxious and depressed.

- She became anti-social.
- She became self-destructive. She engaged in relationships with very abusive men who beat her up.
- She stopped eating regularly and got vitamin and mineral deficiency. She experienced severe nausea and often vomited. She lost a lot of weight.
- She became very emotional. She had emotional outbursts either aggressive or kept crying.
- She developed sleep problems.
- Sometimes she just passed out with a lit cigarette and was not able to wake up. I sometimes thought she had died.
- She became irrational. She gave a man $8500 that she had just met. Over a period of time, she spent the whole inheritance from my father.

- She lost her coordination; she fell several times and was badly hurt.
- She went from being a happy, fun-loving and very caring person to falling apart as a human being.

I isolated myself behind locked down curtains for a long period of time. I was diagnosed with PTSD anxiety, panic attacks, and depression.

I started coping with my anxiety and depression the best I could, but it was still overwhelming from time to time. One day I was at the doctor's office for another reason, and I admitted my symptoms with him. He suggested that I take a depression test; I did.

As he was going through it, he became more and more pale. He suddenly grabbed the phone and said: "I am calling the psychiatric Emergency Room at the hospital to tell them that I am sending you over to them in a taxi, NOW."

It caught me off guard because I just told him that I was trying to cope with my anxiety, panic attacks and depression. He insisted strongly, and I said that I would ride my bike over the psychiatric Emergency Room at the hospital and talk with them.

When I arrived, I was taken to a room where two psychiatrists were sitting at a table. During the 1 ½—2 hours evaluation they did, I told them about my techniques and how the techniques and my daily choices helped me cope with my current situation. I had witnessed my grieving mother falling apart as a human being. Because of that, I chose not to take any pharmaceutical drugs. Suicide was never an option but healing through natural ways was.

Although surprised, they accepted my request to not to be hospitalized, or to take any pharmaceutical medications and instead talk with a psychiatrist who did not prescribe pharmaceutical medications. I then met with the psychiatrist regularly over a couple months. One day she said,"You are doing it, you found your way and you are healing yourself. You don't need me or any medications." I was so happy.

I, myself, chose to start up seeing a Cognitive Behavioral Psychologist so I had someone to reflect with. The Cognitive Behavioral Psychologist was of immense help. I highly recommend seeing a Cognitive Behavioral Psychologist. And then, after a period of time, she said exactly the same as the words. "You are doing it; you found your way and you are healing yourself." You don't need me anymore. I am so happy for you."

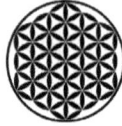

CHAPTER TWENTY-TWO

WHAT DID I DO?

Very often, if not always, anxiety and depression go hand in hand. The anxiety can create depression or depression can create anxiety. Healing one may heal the other. I began to develop my own coping techniques and prayers, which you may find inspiring or even hilarious. The different techniques help increase dopamine, serotonin and endorphins.

FORGIVE YOURSELF

There are heavy stigmas related to addiction, anxiety, and depression. When we are anxious, depressed or using drugs we often feel ashamed and don't feel good enough. We can feel that we have failed as human beings or just feel worthless. When I forgave myself, a heavy burden of shame left and created space for something new.

Under the influence of drugs or in withdrawal, you might have made some pretty bad decisions you are not proud of. Either way, you need to forgive yourself and move on. Don't judge or shame yourself. If you keep pounding yourself, you will feed low self-esteem and shame. You don't need that in a healing and rebuilding process. When you feel better, you can rebalance bad deeds from the past by doing good deeds. You are still a unique human being.

I CHANGED MY DIET

I stopped eating processed food. The majority of vitamins and minerals are destroyed during processing. Instead, I started to cook from scratch, real fresh food or I would eat raw vegetables. I took my time to prepare or cook the food and enjoyed it when I was done. I had my focus on something which was good for me. Sometimes I would go to the beach or the forest and eat there.

EXERCISE

I decided to ride my bike for a period of time, instead of riding the train or bus. I choose my bike for the exercise and fresh air. I started walking to the park for the exercise and to be out among other people. I also started to do exercise regularly at the gym and I went to indoor swimming pools and swam 20 laps, 40 laps, 60 laps, etc. Water is emotion in the magic world, so whenever I was swimming I would let the water wash of any stress, heal and balance my emotions. After swimming I went to a sauna, hot tub, a steam room or a salt pool-whatever they could offer me after a swim. I began to enjoy being in a body. When I was in any shower at any time, I would wash away any negative energy or thoughts from my being. Exercise helped me tremendously to heal. Exercise release endorphins, made me lose weight, got me into really good shape, gave me strength and self-esteem, and helped me to get good sleep.

MUDRA

I noticed that Buddha always sits in meditation with his thumb and index finger together on each individual hand. I found out that this specific mudra (finger gesture) helped me to center and integrate my being. This was especially helpful when I felt out of myself, by myself or overwhelmed by other people or their emotions. I could just put my hands in my pocket or just stand naturally and do the mudra, no one would notice that.

COLORS

Our body has 7 energy wheels called chakras. Each has its own individual color.

We all have a heart chakra and the color is green.

Color is vibration.

It is commonly known that we receive with our left side and we give with our right side. (If you are left-handed you will figure out which side works for you personally).

If I was sitting on a train or bus when a panic attack with rapid heartbeat began, I would look at something green and think that the vibration of the color would go in through my left eye and down to my heart and rebalance my heart/ chakra. Combined with breathing, I would be focused and ride through it within a couple of minutes. Sometimes the fear of a panic attack can ignite a panic attack. The fact that I was able to ride through a panic attack reduced my anxiety and fear of panic attacks.

GROUNDING

Out of my head and into my body. If it is warm enough, it is a great idea to walk barefoot. By feeling my feet connecting to the ground, lying on the ground, or sitting next to a tree was very grounding. Visualize yourself growing roots all the way to the center of the earth.

STOP THE THOUGHT

I would mindfully repeat, "STOP" inside myself, and then redirect my thought towards something I looked forward to doing in the future. This was a great technique which often helped me stop thoughts going in circles.

REDIRECT OR CHANGE YOUR THOUGHT

When you experience a negative or fear-based thought, you can make a conscious choice to change that thought or picture and replace it with the opposite, a positive outcome.

PRAYERS

It doesn't really matter who or what you believe in. For me, God is the creator of the universe. Everything and nothing at all. Eternal and in the present moment of NOW. Love, you, me and all other living beings. When we numb ourselves with drugs, we also disconnect from that source. Praying helped me to reconnect, relax and surrender, knowing there is something greater than me which can help me and it did. I looked at my anxiety and depression as spiritual development; I was learning about myself and was growing as a human being. I still went through the rite of passage or the valley of death, whatever we call it, but I felt protected. I asked God for guidance, healing, and protection.

BREATHING

Breathing. One day I realized that when I was in control of my breathing, I was also in control over a panic attack. In a panic attack, we tend to hyperventilate by breathing fast. When my heart was racing I was able to lower my heart rate by focusing on my breathing. I would take a deep breath and hold my breath for a longer period of time than normal; then I slowly let it out, followed by another deep breath and holding it. Then my heart beat would start going down in tempo and normalize again. Breathing has an impact on dopamine, serotonin and endorphins.

You and I and everyone else are on the earth for a reason. We are all individual and unique; we all have more than one purpose. I found one important purpose: Loving myself- healing me, regenerating me and my being. When I overflow, I will share and help heal other people. That is my second purpose.

FACING MY FEAR BY DOING THE THINGS I WAS AFRAID OF

If I was to take the train or a bus, I would do it, sit down or stand close to the exit and use my techniques, if needed. If shopping or standing in line I would be aware of the exit, if needed, which I sometimes only needed one time to go through. Once in a while I decided to "abort my mission" if I felt it was too overwhelming, but I would do my mission again right after, once or twice, and then succeed. If I didn't succeed the first time, I would stay persistent and do it again until I succeeded. This got much easier the moment I had a couple of techniques like mentioned above.

PARALLEL PROCESS

Some of my daily chores I turned into parallel processes. Taking a shower became relaxing and washing off negative energy. Cleaning up around me became cleaning up inside as well. It was good because in the shadows of depression, people often let go of personal hygiene and cleanliness. Here I turned them into helpful techniques which helped to heal me.

MUSIC IS HEALING

Music made me feel relaxed and I listened to music for hours in the background every day. No, it was not gangster rap or anything else with any negative vibes…. It was positive and uplifting music like instrumental, ambient and cozy Brazilian samba. Only music with positive vibes, listen to it or play music and sing.

MEDITATION/MINDFULNESS IS HEALING

YouTube is amazing when it comes to finding relaxing bi-neural beats, music,and meditations for anxiety, healing and relaxation. Put your headphones on…..

THINK POSITIVE, BE POSITIVE

Focus on positive things and stay away from negative things when you watch TV, read something and listen to music. What you focus on is what you get. I would be happy and celebrate myself when I reached a new goal, even small goals. How did I celebrate myself? I was happy and thankful for each goal I reached, even small ones.

NATURE

Forest, park, beach... It all counts. I would pack a yummy lunch and go to the beach, walk in the park, or go to the forest by myself. Nature is epic. I would go there and just sit down, watch, listen or lie down and listen for a while. Later I would enjoy my lunch. Then I would return home healed and enriched. When I was feeling better with human company, I would introduce my secret spots to friends. Nature is God.

BE THANKFUL FOR WHAT YOU HAVE OR WHAT YOU EXPERIENCE

What you focus on is what you get. If you focus on positive things, you will experience more and more positive things. Very little can go very far. Even being thankful for a flower I saw, the sun shining, a bird I heard or a pleasant smell of spring or the ocean. Everything counts.

SLEEP

I quickly realized that if I was thinking too much at night time, then it helped me a lot to write the things down, or write a list of the things I needed to do. Having a list to follow and check off the tasks when done gave me a good feeling. The same thing in the morning, I would write down what I had experienced in dreamland. Plenty of exercises helped me to sleep better and longer.

INSOMNIA, NIGHTMARES AND SLEEP PARALYSIS

When weaning off an addiction or experiencing anxiety and depression, people often experience insomnia, nightmares or sleep paralysis before falling to sleep, during sleep or early in the morning when waking. I did experience these things and I coped with them.

I distanced myself from the experience. I am not my thoughts, I am witnessing them. I realized that thoughts have a short time span. They could only be there if I gave them feedback by inner comments, and only short term if I didn't. I stopped the thoughts or I redirected them with prayer. If you are religious or believe in God, then prayer is a very strong protector, guide and healer.

Drugs and alcohol are dark and deceitful.

Drugs and alcohol change people's behavior.

Drugs and alcohol make people do evil things.

Under the influence of drugs or alcohol, people often seem to change their behavior sometimes like being possessed. I took the perspective that insomnia, nightmares and sleep paralysis are related to dark spirits fighting to get me to start using substances to numb myself, and they were fighting not to leave me. Then I distanced myself and I became a witness. It then became less intense. My mantra was: This is very unpleasant and it is temporary. My internal prayer was: Dear God, please protect me, guide me and heal me. Shine your light upon me, from inside out and fill this room, I love you. And yes, praying in the darkest hour helps. Even if you don't believe in God, try a prayer next time; I might actually help you anyway.

I had several periods where I experienced sleep paralysis. (Waking up and not being able to move, experiencing suffocating while having the feeling there is something bad or evil energy in the room). The first times I experienced it, I was terrified. Then I used my prayer, not fighting to move and I would stay calm instead of going into a panic. It would disappear shortly after. I later noticed that it only happened when I was sleeping on my back. This is where the word nightmare actually comes from. A mare (demon) sitting on the chest, suffocating and giving bad dreams at night. If I experience sleep paralysis today, I just say a prayer and turn on my side and continue to sleep.

Sleeping on your side with a pillow between your legs will greatly reduce sleep paralysis if not eliminate it 100%.

I experienced insomnia, nightmares, and sleep paralysis and I coped with them. Exercise made me tired at night time, healthy food rebalanced my body, mind, and spirit, techniques helped during my healing, prayers and over-the-counter sleep supplements like Kava and Valerian helped me relax and sleep better.

SPIRITUAL GROUP OR SUPPORT GROUP

Using drugs impact both the body and the mind. When we use drugs, pharmaceuticals, and alcohol, we numb ourselves from reality, feelings and emotions. When we stop using, we start feeling and sensing reality around us again. If we have been numb for a long time, it can almost be as if we have to learn how to start living again. Always keep in mind that there are self-help groups or support groups with like-minded people who understand what you are experiencing.

It can also be any spiritual group like Christian, Catholic, Sufi, Hindu etc. I myself was introduced to one with no specific religious preferences. Open Heart Tribe, all were welcome which was perfect. It was a great mix of everything. God is everything.

SHARING

Every time we met, we took the time to share whatever we wanted. What made it a difficult week or what made it an awesome week. All were welcome, people did not have to share their deepest and most vulnerable self. If over time any sensitive things like that were shared, it was embraced and not judged. Everyone there was accepted and if anyone couldn't behave, they would find the way out themselves. Cut loose and let go. Sharing was a great learner for me, I shared and it released energy. Over time I ended up not caring about being judged. Eventually the fear of being judged was just a thought in me, maybe not real at all, and if any judge me, then it tells more about them than me. And after all, carrying loads of things around just drags us down.

CONTACT EXERCISES

We did contact exercises where we moved around in a circle meeting and greeting each other, or we just sat in front of each other and looking into each other eyes, connecting with each other. This was a great help for me to start connecting with other people again and feel them.

MEDITATION

From time to time we would do meditations. Either shorter ones by ourselves or longer ones, guided meditations. This was great help for me toward starting meditation on my own which I have done for years now.

DANCE

We would usually spend time dancing to a couple of tunes. High and energetic or just slow and meditative with closed eyes. It didn't matter how it looked or how good we were at dancing, and people didn't really care at all. It was all about body movement and being present. It helped me to get into rhythm, appreciate my body again and enjoy using it.

SING

From time to time we would sing. Some of the songs were spiritual mantras and others just because they were positive songs. Language or songs didn't really matter. The intention behind the song mattered. It helped me to communicate again and not being anxious of hearing my own voice speak out loud.

BODY CONTACT

We did body contact exercises like touching each other very gently with respect for boundaries, and exercises where we gently massaged each other on top of our clothes with respect for personal areas. People and especially children can die from lack of body contact. The lack of body contact after being isolated for a couple years was what made me send out a wish for a group like this. I realized my lack of body contact and how much I needed it to survive.

AMAZING FRIENDSHIPS

During this time, I formed new amazing friendships. That is what we need to thrive. Authentic friends who want the best for us are necessary to thrive as human beings. These friends I still have today, 15 years later.

MEN'S GROUP

Over time it led some of us to form a women's group and a men's group. David Deida (a well-known couples and relationship therapist) inspired us. In our men's group, we met every week for 5 years before I had to let go of it and the group is still alive today, 9 years later.

The right food, exercise and being a part of a spiritual group helped me to regenerate my physical, emotional, mental and spiritual being. It helped me to connect with people and build new long-lasting relationships. I developed courage, motivation, self-confidence, trust, strength, happiness, harmony and the ability to give and receive love and compassion. I went from being anxious, sad and depressive to optimistic and positive. I became stronger than I had ever been before. I healed without any pharmaceutical medication. Step by step, I found my way through, and so can you.

Shortly after my way through "The Valley of Death" and still coping with anxiety and depression, I attended a university and achieved a bachelor's degree in Social Science. I later passed an international therapist training.

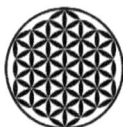

CHAPTER TWENTY-THREE

NEVER GIVE UP

I f you go down the road to relapse for a short period of time, (which hopefully you won't, however it might happen to some people), then keep the following in mind: you will regret it because it is not worth it, and it can throw you into full addiction again. If you do the same quantum of drugs as you did before you weaned off, you might actually overdose and die. That is not worth it either.

It is likely you won't experience the same drug experience, physical, mental or emotional as you did in the past.

If you do it anyway, then forgive yourself and move on. Wean off again right away.

Remember when you go through a hard time that triggers, emotional roller coasters related to PAWS are right around the corner! Rome was not built in one day. Keep in mind that drugs have messed big time with your natural chemistry of your brain. Your natural dopamine, serotonin, endorphins and vitamin and minerals levels may be pretty imbalanced. It will take time to rebalance these levels, maybe even up 6 months to a year depending on your efforts. Don't let that trick you, eventually if you want to wean off an addiction you will have to go through the process now or later. It is well worth taking the fight and come through to the other side. There is light at the end of the tunnel.

Throughout this book, you have been introduced to the many tools which can make this a successful experience for you. A second chance. Use the tools and take one day at a time, even an hour or a minute, if that is needed.

Be thankful that you came through the first couple of weeks. The first couple of weeks are the worst. Remember the insane hell of initial withdrawal is what keeps many people addicted on prescription medication and maintenance drugs for many years, for some people the rest of their life.

Let your mantra be: "Right now it is unpleasant; it is a part of the process and it is temporary." You may have children, parents, siblings, friends or maybe a dog. Even start with the small things in life. Raindrops on your face, a flower blooming, a nice smell, a stranger or a child smiling, the wind in the trees, a light ray, waves coming into shore…… Be patient, work your way through it. Over time you will notice a difference, and your life will get better. Much better. Be thankful for what you have, it can all be gone in a split second. You don't want that.

Look one year ahead of you and see how your brain chemistry is rebalanced, you are happy now because you got a second chance and a new life. Your body is detoxed, you eat healthy, you exercise regularly, you have new friends, a job or maybe you are achieving the education you always wanted. Maybe life gave you a new perspective and new strengths. You are loved and you can feel love and compassion again. Life is beautiful.

This is what you want to create for your future and hold on to: that when you are having a hard time, you can do it. Those who can wean off drugs are heroes. You can be one of them.

> *"I got clean September 2016 off Oxy's. Had been on them for over 10 years. It was like losing my best worst friend. Was taking 8 to 12 30 mgs a day destroying cars, relationships, family and myself. I'm so sorry you had to lose so much to get where you are, but unfortunately that's the unwritten rule of this roller coaster ride..... If you make it out alive. Now is the beginning of the rest of your life. Stay clean and stay strong." (HC).*

> *"First there is sickness, then pain, then despair. But when sadness comes it is almost a relief because you have not felt any emotion for a loooong time. Then comes the good ones, laughter, love, motivation..... And you thank yourself because in the end it was worth the fight after all...." (JS).*

YOU GOT THIS!

ARTICLE, VIDEO AND BOOK REFERENCES:

Testimonies and sources in this book are from private internet groups. These groups are private because of the stigma related to drug abuse. Many of the people in these groups are ordinary people who have lives, family and study or work. Their spouse, children, family, co-workers and friends may have absolutely no idea that these people are former users, hence them being in a private group. I respect keeping them private and protecting themselves and their lives, which is why they are in a private group and I honor that and I will not reveal anyone. No one shall have their life exposed or destroyed by being outed for the personal experiences they share from the heart to help other people in need. They are heroes. Big heroes. If you want another 100+ pages of public Kratom testimonies please go to American Kratom Association or look up the 8-Factor Analysis of the last 100 pages.

The 8 factor analysis. Assessment of Kratom under the CSA eight Factors and Scheduling Recommendation. Pinney Associates 2016. https://docs.wixstatic.com/ugd/9ba5da_5a326244df824bc984121783fdc4a65c.pdf

Neurobiology of Kratom and its main alkaloid Mitragynine. Kumarnsit et al. 2007 and Idayu et al. 2011. http://uthscsa.edu/artt/AddictionJC/KratomReview.pdf

Mitragynina Speciosa leaf extract exhibits antipsychotic effect. https://www.ncbi.nlm.nih.gov/pmc/articles/PMC5138496/

Update on the Pharmacology and legal Status of Kratom. Walter C. Prozialeck, PhD 2016. http://jaoa.org/article.aspx?articleid=2588524

Drugs A-Z List Various side effects etc. https://www.rxlist.com/drugs/alpha_a.htm

Drugs A-Z List Various side effects etc. https://www.webmd.com/drugs/2/index

https://www.rxlist.com/Benzodiazepines-page2/drugs-condition.htm

Kratom presentation 2017. Dr. Oliver Grundman College of Pharmacy, University of Florida. https://www.youtube.com/watch?v=Yehuz5HmOGs

Dr. Tom O'Brien.ei/100 Kratom facts.

https://www.organicfacts.net/health-benefits/other/Kratom-leaves.html

http://Kratomguides.com/top-15-health-benefits-of-Kratom/

https://www.iloveKratom.com/Kratom-forum/general-dialogue/3872-the-real-truth-about-yellow-gold-bentuangie-Kratom-by-joe-sokol

Self-treatment of Opioid withdrawal using Kratom. (Mitragynia Speciosa Korth). Boyer et al. 2008, https://www.ncbi.nlm.nih.gov/pmc/articles/PMC3670991/.

https://www.inquisitr.com/opinion/4659908/fda-Kratom-advisory-unfounded-foia-docs-show/

Kratom exposures reported to poison centers US 2010-2015. Warner et al 2016. https://www.cdc.gov/mmwr/volumes/65/wr/pdfs/mm6529a4.pdf

A drug fatality involving Kratom? https://www.ncbi.nlm.nih.gov/m/pubmed/23082895/

FOIA shows FDA's data on Kratom deaths are lies and complete propaganda. http://thefreethoughtproject.com/Kratom-deaths-fda-bllsht/?utm_medium=pushnotifyandutm_source=browserandutm_campaign=pushfeedsandutm_content=push

The scheduling of Kratom and selective use of data. Griffen et al. 2016. https://www.ncbi.nlm.nih.gov/labs/articles/28937941/

Experiences of Kratom Users: A Qualitative Analysis. Swogger et al 2015. http://blogs.ubc.ca/walshlab/files/2015/06/Kratom.pdf

Haveman-Reinicke 2011, http://www.europsy-journal.com/article/S0924-9338(11)71761-8/pdf, Dr. Tom O'Brien.ie.

Antidepressants, Antipsychotics, and Stimulants by Dr. David W. Tanton, Ph.D

US National Library of Medicine National Institutes of Health.

https://www.drugabuse.gov.

Charlotte Gerson: Healing the Gerson way. Defeating cancer and other chronic diseases.

10 benefits of coffee enemas. Patricia Ramos, healthyhints.com 2017.

Katie young, honeycolony.com 2016

https://www.ncbi.nlm.nih.gov/pmc/articles/PMC4241367/

http://www.webmd.com

https://www.ncbi.nlm.nih.gov/pmc/articles/PMC3560823/

Pharmacology Chapter 22 Anticonvulsants, and Agents for Alzheimer's Disease. https://quizlet.com/45252742/pharmacology-chapter-22-anticonvulsantsand-agents-for-alzheimers-disease-flash-cards/

https://www.ncbi.nlm.nih.gov/pubmed/23673774

https://www.psychologistworld.com/biological/neurotransmitters/dopamine

https://www.news-medical.net/health/What-is-Dopamine.aspx

https://www.medicalnewstoday.com/kc/serotonin-facts-232248

https://www.webmd.com/depression/features/serotonin#1

https://science.howstuffworks.com/life/endorphins.htm

https://www.macalester.edu/academics/psychology/whathap/ubnrp/meth08/biochemistry/serotonin.htm

https://www.medicinenet.com/endorpnins

https://draxe.com/what-are-endorphins/

https://www.rodalewellness.com/health/breathing-exercises

https://bebrainfit.com/increase-endorphins/

https://www.livestrong.com/article/185758-how-to-balance-dopamine-and-serotonin-levels/

https://helloendless.com/10-ways-to-increase-dopamine-to-boost-your-productivity/

https://www.healthline.com/nutrition/magnesium-deficiency-symptoms

https://www.webmd.com/vitamins-supplements/ingredientmono-1037-tyrosine.aspx?activeingredientid=1037&

https://www.sclfhacked.com/blog/tyrosine-8-proven-health-benefits-tyrosine/

https://www.optimallivingdynamics.com/blog/7-important-nutrients-depleted-by-psychiatric-drugs antidepressants-antipsychotics-stimulants-Benzodiazepines-induced-guide-vitamins-medications

https://www.health.harvard.edu/staying-healthy/foods-that-fight-inflammation

http://www.eatthis.com/anti-inflammatory-foods/

B 12 deficiency: https://www.ncbi.nlm.nih.gov/pmc/articles/PMC3271502/

http://lpi.oregonstate.edu/mic/minerals/magnesium

Zinc: https://www.ncbi.nlm.nih.gov/pubmed/23567517

CoQ10: https://www.ncbi.nlm.nih.gov/pubmed/25603363

Vitamin D: http://glutathionepro.com/how-to-treat-depression-with-nutrition/

https://www.healthline.com/nutrition/candida-symptoms-treatment

https://www.livestrong.com/article/385118-vitamins-minerals-in-coffee/

https://www.healthline.com/nutrition/top-13-evidence-based-health-benefits-of-coffee#section13

DLPA: https://liftmode.com/mood-lifting/phenylalanine.html#_ftn3, https://www.ncbi.nlm.nih.gov/pubmed/335027, http://www.uofmhealth.org/health-library/hn-2895002.

Therapeutic effects of Cannabis and cannabinoids.(https://www.ncbi.nlm.nih.gov/books/NBK425767/)

Warner et al 2016, Dr. Tom O'Brien.ie.

Boyer https://www.ncbi.nlm.nih.gov/pubmed/18482427.

John P. Cunha, DO, Facoep. & Rxlist.com 2017.

European Monitoring Center for Drugs and Drug Addiction.

http://www.emcdda.europa.eu/publications/drug-profiles

C Ulbricht et al. J Diet Suppl 10 (2), 152-170. 6 2013.

http://www.stltoday.com/lifestyles/health-med-fit/health/
to-your-good-health/do-calcium-channel-blockers-block-
calcium-supplements/article_49dfb084-f9bc-5da7-8b59-
fd0b970d0ebd.html

https://www.americanKratom.org

http://speciosa.org/home/Kratom-legality-map

https://www.accessdata.fda.gov/scripts/
InteractiveNutritionFactsLabel/factsheets/Vitamin_and_
Mineral_Chart.pdf

https://www.theatlantic.com/health/archive/2017/06/nejm-
letter-opioids/528840/

https://www.scribd.com/doc/164400341/The-Complete-
Ashton-Manual-Works-PDF

The Benzodiazepine Medical Disaster—Benzo Xanax
Klonopin Valium Ativan Documentary (52:12). https://www.
youtube.com/watch?v=NovJdBu-A2M

One nation overdosed. Documentary (44:40). https://www.
youtube.com/watch?v=S9KRdqwQcdo

Dead by Fentanyl. Documentary.

Dr. Nancy White. Why antidepressants are dangerous. https://
www.youtube.com/watch?v=Ik0RTsIAEBU

Psychiatrist MD. Peter Breggin. Psychiatric drugs are more dangerous than you ever imagined. https://www.youtube.com/watch?v=luKsQaj0hzs

Dr. Gary Kolhs. What natural products work as antidepressants. https://www.youtube.com/watch?v=zSWoW2bPo08

Psychiatrist MD. Peter Breggin. Antidepressants & suicide—Congressional testimony before the Veterans Affairs Committee 2010. https://www.youtube.com/watch?v=SBJfZtB_3cc

https://www.psychologytoday.com/blog/obsessively-yours/201001/five-reasons-not-take-ssris

https://breggin.com/the-proven-dangers-of-antidepressants/

https://www.drugs.com/drug-class/ssri-antidepressants.html

http://www.rcpsych.ac.uk/healthadvice/treatmentsandwellbeing/antidepressants/comingoffantidepressants.aspx6

https://www.therecoveryvillage.com/Benzodiazepine-addiction/Benzodiazepine-taper/#gref

https://www.therecoveryvillage.com/opiate-addiction/opiate-taper/#gref

https://www.optimallivingdynamics.com/blog/7-important-nutrients-depleted-by-psychiatric-drugs-antidepressants-antipsychotics-stimulants-Benzodiazepines-induced-guide-vitamins-medications

Gabapentin/Nerontin:

1). https://www.youtube.com/watch?v=vRbFuVwqlsg

2). https://www.youtube.com/watch?v=xFv_Uqv5jXw

AED taper. https://www.medscape.com/viewarticle/513638

https://www.benzo.org.uk/pws04.htm

Lorazepam. https://www.youtube.com/watch?v=OQIHiRnIcck

Gabapentin. https://www.youtube.com/watch?v=mFD9Y1ib36s&t=28s

Celexa. https://www.youtube.com/watch?v=lx_Zr9q6TP4

SSRIs and their side effects. https://www.youtube.com/watch?v=fIyc9QWvUhY

http://speciosa.org/home/Kratom-legality-map.

https://www.botanical-education.org/wp-content/uploads/2017/01/Dr.-Jane-IP-Synergy-Kratom-Comment.pdf

http://www.americankratom.org/images/file/Document%2012%20FDA%20Fails%20to%20Follow%20the%20Science%20-%20Babin%20-%20August%202018.pdf

https://www.cchrint.org/pdfs/violence-report.pdf

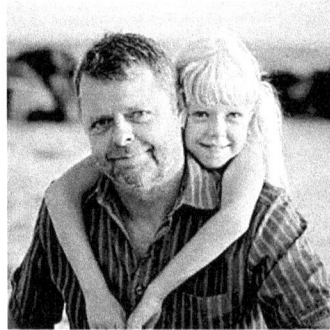

Dan Knudsen was born in 1968, raised and educated in Denmark. He graduated his Bachelor Summa Cum laude as a Social worker, Bac. Soc. Paed. He personally experienced the devastating effects of addiction in his family and among friends. Due to intense personal life experiences he was diagnosed with PTSD. Anxiety, panic attacks and depression. He worked himself through the PTSD without taking any pharmaceutical prescription medication. In the self help book he shares his personal experiences of how he worked himself through anxiety, panic attacks and depression. He later did a therapist training.

www.ingramcontent.com/pod-product-compliance
Lightning Source LLC
Chambersburg PA
CBHW060323030426
42336CB00011B/1177